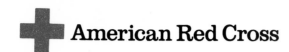

American Red Cross

Marian

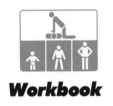

Workbook

American Red Cross Community CPR

ISBN 0-86536-083-9

Acknowledgments

This course is based on the Standards and Guidelines established by the 1985 National Conference on Cardiopulmonary Resuscitation and Emergency Cardiac Care.

The course and this workbook are products of the 1987–1988 CPR/First Aid Project at American Red Cross national headquarters. Unit One of the workbook is composed of Chapters 3 through 6 of the *American Red Cross: Adult CPR* workbook. Those chapters were prepared by American Red Cross staff, volunteers, and consultants as acknowledged in the *American Red Cross: Adult CPR* workbook (Stock No. 329128, Feb. 1987).

The development team for this course and for Unit Two of the workbook included M. Elizabeth Buoy, M.P.H.; Valerie W. Drake, M.A.; Lawrence Newell, Ed.D.; Suzanne M. Randolph, Ph.D.; and Sarah A. Snyder, M.A.T. Additional assistance was provided by Program Development Division staff including Bruce Spitz, director; Frank Carroll; Jessica Bernstein, M.P.H.; Karen Peterson, Ph.D.; Victoria Scott, M.P.A.; Pamela B. Mangu, M.A.; and Susan Walter. The following national sector staff also provided assistance: Joan Handler; Alfred J. Katz, M.D.; Carole Kauffman, R.N.; John M. Malatak, M.S.; and Donald Miller, J.D.

Technical advice and review were provided by:

Susan Aronson, M.D., F.A.A.P., Practicing Pediatrician, Clinical Professor of Pediatrics, Hahnemann University, Philadelphia, Pa.

Allan Braslow, Ph.D., Faculty, 1985 National Conference on CPR and Emergency Cardiac Care; Braslow & Associates.

Daniel L. Cavallaro, NREMT, Assistant in Surgery, Division of Cardiothoracic Surgery, Clinical Instructor of Medicine, University of South Florida College of Medicine, Tampa, Fla.

Leon Chameides, M.D., Director of Pediatric Cardiology, and Clinical Professor of Pediatrics, University of Connecticut Health Center, Hartford Hospital.

Richard Christoph, M.D., Emergency Medical Services Department, University of Virginia Medical Center, Charlottesville, Va.

Sandra E. Clarke, S.C.C., Executive Director, Advanced Coronary Treatment (ACT) Foundation of Canada, Ottawa, Ont.

Douglas D'Arnall, U.S. Lifesaving Association Representative to the Council for National Cooperation in Aquatics, Beach Services Manager, Huntington Beach, Calif.

George L. Foltin, M.D., F.A.A.P., Director, Pediatric Emergency Services, Bellevue Hospital Center, and Assistant Professor of Pediatrics, New York University School of Medicine.

Rene Michalski, EMT-P, Paramedic Instructor/ Coordinator, McLennan Community College, Continuing Education Division, Waco, Tex.

Marisa Mize, R.N., M.S.N., Catholic University of America, School of Nursing, Washington, D.C.

William J. Schneiderman, Adjunct Clinical Instructor, Emergency Care Institute, NYU/Bellevue Hospital Center, and former Education Coordinator, Department of Emergency Medical Services, New York Infirmary-Beekman Downtown Hospital.

Michael G. Tunik, M.D., Attending Physician in Clinical Pediatrics, Bellevue Hospital Center, and Instructor in Clinical Pediatrics, New York University School of Medicine.

Mark D. Widome, M.D., Chairman, Committee on Accident and Poison Prevention, American Academy of Pediatrics, Hershey, Pa.

This manuscript was also reviewed by the National Academy of Sciences–National Research Council Committee to Advise the American National Red Cross.

Field representatives providing advice and guidance through the 1987–1988 Red Cross CPR Advisory Committee included:

W. Larry Bair, Central Iowa Chapter, Des Moines, Iowa

D. Earl Harbert, Field Service Manager, Wichita, Kan.

Jerry Hummel, Southeastern Michigan Chapter, Detroit, Mich.

Lonnie Kirby, Western Operations Headquarters, Burlingame, Calif.

Wanda Leffler, Indianapolis Area Chapter, Indianapolis, Ind.

Mary M. "Posie" Mansfield, Danvers, Mass.; Chair, Basic Life Support Sub-Committee of the CPR Advisory Committee.

C. Ray McLain, R.N., M.S.N., Assistant Professor, University of Alabama, Birmingham, Ala.; Chairman, Infant/Child CPR Sub-Committee of the CPR Advisory Committee.

Marshall Meyer, Oregon Trail Chapter, Portland, Oreg.

Gary J. Taylor, Greater Kansas City Chapter, Kansas City, Mo.

Richard Tulis, American Red Cross of Massachusetts Bay, Boston, Mass.

John Wagner, Albany Area Chapter, Albany, N.Y.

Acknowledgments

Red Cross chapters that participated in field tests
included:

    Arlington County Chapter, Arlington, Va.
    Indianapolis Area Chapter, Indianapolis, Ind.
    Midway-Kansas Chapter, Wichita, Kan.
    Oregon Trail Chapter, Portland, Oreg.
    Pasadena Chapter, Pasadena, Calif.

Contents

Contents

Why the American Red Cross Teaches This Course

The American Red Cross has designed this course to teach you lifesaving skills to use in respiratory and cardiac emergencies. A respiratory emergency is a situation (such as near-drowning or choking) that makes it difficult or impossible for a person to breathe. A cardiac emergency occurs when the heart is not working properly or when the heart stops beating.

A respiratory or cardiac emergency can happen to an adult, to a child, or to an infant. This course will help you learn about these emergencies and how to give first aid, whether the victim is an adult, a child, or an infant. Your desire to learn this information and important lifesaving skills will help you succeed in this course.

For adults over the age of 45, heart disease is the leading cause of death. This year about a million and a half people in the United States will have a heart attack. One third of these people will die. This means that about 1,500 people die every day from heart attacks.

One out of every two people in the United States can expect to die from a heart attack or a related disease of the blood vessels. This is an important national problem.

Most people who die from a heart attack die before they get to a hospital. Some people survive a heart attack because a bystander trained in the skills taught in this course knows what to do and because the community has an emergency medical services (EMS) system to give advanced medical care at the scene of the emergency.

Another important national problem is the number of children killed and injured in accidents. More than 8,000 children under 14 years of age die of injuries each year in the United States. Injury from accidents is the leading cause of death for children ages one through 14. For infants under one year of age, injury is one of the four leading causes of death. You could be the one to prevent a life-threatening injury by reducing the risk of injury. This course will help you make a plan you can use to prevent injuries to children and infants.

When a respiratory or cardiac emergency does happen—for example, when a child chokes or an infant suffocates—you could be the one to help save that child or infant by giving first aid until advanced emergency medical care arrives.

This course will teach you—
1. How to give first aid for choking and other respiratory emergencies.
2. How to recognize when someone needs CPR.
3. How to give CPR to someone whose heart has stopped.
4. How to use the emergency medical services (EMS) system.
5. How to reduce the risk of dying from a heart attack.
6. How to recognize the signals of a heart attack and give first aid to reduce the chance that the victim's heart will stop.
7. How to reduce the risk of injury to children and infants.

In the first part of this course, you will learn lifesaving skills to help adults. You can use these adult skills to help a person nine years of age or older. In the second part of the course, you will learn lifesaving skills to help a child age one through eight. You will then learn skills to help an infant less than one year old.

The materials for the course are described below.

Workbook

This workbook is structured to help you get the most out of the course. Both the workbook and the course are divided into two units. Unit One focuses on first aid for respiratory and cardiac emergencies in adults. Unit Two highlights prevention of childhood injury and focuses on first aid for respiratory and cardiac emergencies in children and infants.

Objectives

Each chapter in this workbook begins with a list of objectives. The objectives tell you what you should be able to do when you finish the course activities for that chapter.

Review Questions

There are review questions in each chapter. Answer the questions to check how well you are learning and to prepare for the final test. Write your answers in the workbook. The correct answers follow each group of review questions, so be sure to go back and correct any wrong answers.

Skill Sheets

Some chapters have skill sheets that tell how to do certain first aid skills. The skill sheets also have pictures to help you understand and follow the directions on the skill sheets. Use the skill sheets when you practice the skills that are shown to you in this course. You will practice on a partner and on manikins.

Glossary

There is a glossary at the end of this book to explain words that you may not know.

Film/Video

You will see short films. These films show real-life situations in which you would use the skills you learned in the course. These films show you the skills that you will practice. Watching the films closely will help you do well when you practice.

Tests

There are two kinds of tests in this course: skill tests and a written test. You will take a skill test after you have practiced each skill and you are ready to be tested. You will take a written test at the end of the course. It is a multiple-choice test about things you have learned in the course.

Some Health Precautions and Guidelines to Follow During This Course

Infection and Disease

Since the beginning of citizen training in CPR (cardiopulmonary resuscitation), the American Red Cross and the American Heart Association have trained more than 50 million people in these lifesaving skills. According to the Centers for Disease Control (CDC), there has never been a documented case of any infectious disease transmitted through the use of CPR manikins.

The Red Cross follows widely accepted guidelines for the cleaning and decontamination of training manikins. **If these guidelines are consistently followed, and basic personal hygiene (for example, frequent hand-washing) is practiced, the risk of any kind of disease transmission during CPR training is extremely low.**

There are also some **health precautions** and guidelines that you should know. You should take these precautions if you have an acute or chronic infection or have a condition that would increase your risk or the other participants' risk of exposure to infections. Most acute infections or conditions, such as a cold, a cut on the hand, or breaks in the skin in or around the mouth, are short-lived. The safest and most practical thing to do if you have an acute infection or condition is to postpone CPR training until, for instance, your cut or abrasion heals, or your cold or influenza is over.

Other infections and conditions may be chronic, or require a longer recovery period, making it impractical to postpone CPR training. In this instance, for your safety and the safety of others, it may be appropriate for you to use a separate manikin for CPR training, after you have discussed your participation with your private physician.

You should **postpone** participation in CPR training if you—
- Have a respiratory infection, such as a cold or a sore throat.
- Believe or know you have recently been exposed to any infection, to which you may be susceptible.
- Are showing signs and symptoms of any infectious disease such as a cold, chicken pox, or mumps, or if you have a fever.
- Have any cuts or sores on your hands, or in or around your mouth (for example, cold sores or recent tooth extraction).
- Know you are seropositive (have had a positive blood test) for hepatitis B surface antigen (HBsAg), indicating that you are currently infected with hepatitis B virus.*

You should request a **separate manikin** if you—
- Know you have a chronic infection such as indicated by long-term seropositivity (long-term positive blood tests) for hepatitis B surface antigen (HBsAg)* or a positive test for anti-HIV (that is, a positive test for anti-bodies to HIV, the virus that causes AIDS).
- Have an acute infection or condition but are unable to postpone CPR training.
- Have a type of condition that makes you unusually susceptible to infection.

If, after you read and consider the above information, you decide that you need to have your own manikin, ask your instructor if one can be made available for your use. If you qualify under the above conditions for the use of a separate manikin, you should discuss this with your instructor, but you will not be required to provide details in your request. The manikin will not be used by anyone else until it has been cleaned according to the recommended end-of-class decontamination procedures. The Red Cross will do its best to provide you with a separate manikin. However, please understand that it may be impossible to do so, especially on short notice, because of limited numbers of manikins for class use. In this instance, you may wish to reschedule CPR training for a later date. The more advance notice you provide, the more likely it is that the Red Cross will be able to accommodate your request.

Guidelines to Follow During Training

To protect yourself and other participants from infection, you should do the following:

- Wash your hands thoroughly before working with the manikin and repeat handwashing as often as is necessary or appropriate.
- Do not eat, drink, use tobacco products, or chew gum immediately before or during manikin use.
- Before you use the manikin, dry the manikin's face with a clean gauze pad. Next, vigorously wipe the manikin's face and the inside of its mouth with a clean gauze pad soaked with either a solution of liquid chlorine bleach and water (sodium hypochlorite and water) or rubbing alcohol. Place this wet pad over the manikin's mouth and nose and wait at least 30 seconds. Then wipe the face dry with a clean gauze pad.
- When practicing what to do for an obstructed airway, simulate (pretend to do) the finger sweep.

Physical Stress and Injury

CPR requires strenuous activity. If you have a medical condition or disability that will prevent you from taking part in the practice sessions, please let your instructor know.

Damage to Manikins

In order to protect the manikins from damage, you should do the following before you begin to practice:

- Remove pens and pencils from your pockets.
- Remove all jewelry.
- Remove lipstick and excess makeup.
- Remove chewing gum and candy from your mouth.

---

*A person with hepatitis B infection will test positive for the hepatitis B surface antigen (HBsAg). Most persons infected with hepatitis B will get better within a period of time. However, some hepatitis B infections will become chronic and will linger for much longer. These persons will continue to test positive for HBsAg, and their decision to participate in CPR training should be guided by their physician.

After a person has had an acute hepatitis B infection, he or she will no longer test positive for the surface antigen but will test positive for the hepatitis B antibody (anti-HBs). Persons who have been vaccinated for hepatitis B will also test positive for the hepatitis antibody. A positive test for the hepatitis B antibody (anti-HBs) should not be confused with a positive test for the hepatitis B surface antigen (HBsAg).

1 How to Deal With an Emergency (Emergency Action Principles)

Adult   9 yrs older
Child   1-9 yrs.
Infant - less 1 yr.

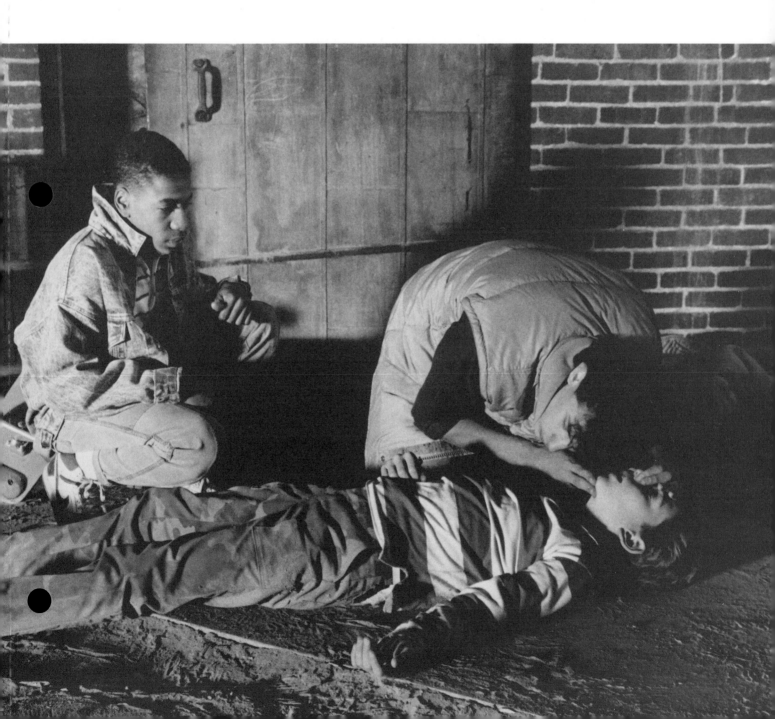

*This workbook will tell you what to do for respiratory emergencies, choking, heart attack, and cardiac arrest. You will also learn how you can prevent some of these emergencies from happening. Before you learn about first aid for these emergencies, you should know certain principles that you should follow in every emergency situation. These are called the **emergency action principles**, and they are discussed in this chapter.*

Objectives

By the time you finish reading this chapter, you should be able to do the following:

1. *List the four emergency action principles (steps you should take in every emergency).*
2. *Explain why you should follow the same steps in every emergency situation.*
3. *Give two reasons why you should identify yourself as a rescuer.*
4. *Describe the purpose and steps of a **primary survey.***
5. *Explain why you should finish a primary survey before phoning the emergency medical services (EMS) system for help.*
6. *List at least four important facts you should give an EMS dispatcher when phoning for help.*
7. *Describe the purpose and steps of a **secondary survey.***
8. *Explain why you should ask a conscious victim's permission before giving first aid.*
9. *Explain when you should get permission before giving first aid to a child or an infant.*

Emergency Action Principles

This chapter gives you a four-step plan of action to use in an emergency. The steps—the emergency action principles—are the same whether the victim is an adult, a child, or an infant. Follow these steps so you don't forget anything that might affect personal safety (yours and the victim's) and the victim's survival. Always do the steps in the order given below. The rest of the chapter will explain more about them.

1. Survey the scene.
2. Do a primary survey of the victim.
3. Call the emergency medical services (EMS) system for help.
4. Do a secondary survey of the victim.

To see why you need to know the emergency action principles, think about this: *You are at home watching television when you hear a cry from outside. You run outside and see a child lying face-down on the side of the road.*

What should you do?

Most people would run straight to the child. But think first. Is there anything wrong with doing that? Is there something you might miss if you ran straight to the child? Look around quickly for someone who was with the child and who could tell you what happened. Is there a parent nearby?

Could the situation be dangerous to you or others nearby? Could there be someone else who is more seriously hurt? A quick look around might give you an idea of what happened.

If you run straight to the child and start to deal with the first problem you see, many things could go wrong. You could get injured, too. You could be hit by a car or injured in some other way. Also, you might not notice others who are hurt.

Review Questions

Check the best answer or fill in the blanks with the right number.

1. Why is it important to follow the same basic steps in every emergency?
   - ☐ a. So that you don't forget anything that might affect personal safety (yours and the victim's) and the victim's survival.
   - ☐ b. So that you will be able to give a complete medical history to the EMS personnel who come to help.
   - ☐ c. So that bystanders will know exactly what you are doing.

2. Put the following four steps of the emergency action principles in the right order.

   Order

   _3_ Phone the EMS system for help.

   _1_ Survey the scene.

   _2_ Do a primary survey of the victim.

   _4_ Do a secondary survey of the victim.

Answers

1. **a.** It is important to follow the same steps in every emergency **so that you don't forget anything that might affect personal safety (yours and the victim's) and the victim's survival.**

2. Emergency action principles—correct order:
   3. Phone the EMS system for help.
   1. Survey the scene.
   2. Do a primary survey of the victim.
   4. Do a secondary survey of the victim.

Survey the Scene

When you hear a call for help, there are certain things that you should always do. As you go to the victim, take in the whole picture. Don't look only at the victim. Take a look all around the victim. This should take only a few seconds and should not delay your caring for the victim. Here are the things to look for:

- **Is the scene safe?** Is the area safe enough for you to approach the victim? For example, is there an exposed electric wire? Are there harmful fumes? Is there danger from passing vehicles? Once you reach the victim, decide if it is safe for you and the victim to stay where you are. Unless you or the victim is in immediate danger from a hazard at the scene, such as leaking gas or fire, don't move the victim.

- **What happened?** What really happened? Look around for clues to tell you the kind of injuries the victim might have. The scene itself often gives you some answers *(Fig. 1)*. If a person is lying next to a ladder, you might assume that he or she has fallen off the ladder and might have broken some bones. An electric wire on the ground next to the victim might mean that the victim has received an electric shock. This information is important, especially when the victim is unconscious and cannot tell you what is wrong and there are no bystanders to give you information.

- **How many people are injured?** Look beyond the victim you see at first glance. There may be other victims. One person may be screaming in pain while another, who may be more seriously injured, is unnoticed because he or she is unconscious. In an auto accident, car doors that are open may mean that there are more victims nearby who were thrown out of or walked from the car.

- **Are there bystanders who can help?** If there are people nearby, use them to help you find out what happened. Maybe someone saw what happened. If a bystander knows the victim, ask if the victim has any medical problems. This information can help you figure out what is wrong with the victim. Bystanders can also phone for help.

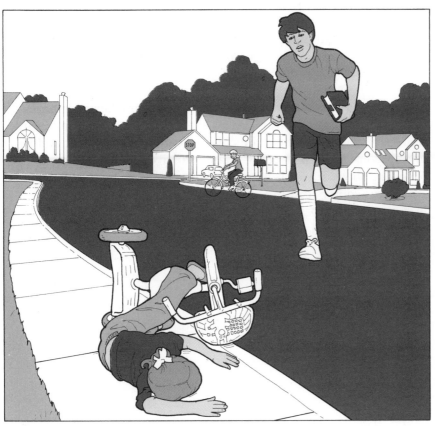

Figure 1
Survey the Scene

Identify Yourself as a Trained Rescuer

Tell the victim and bystanders who you are and that you are trained in first aid. This may help to comfort the victim. It may also help you to take charge of the situation and let someone who may already be caring for the victim know that you are trained in first aid and can help.

Before giving first aid to a person who is conscious, it is important that you ask permission to help the person. Legally, the person must give consent to your offer to give help. If the person is unconscious, consent is implied. This means that the law assumes that an unconscious victim would have given consent if conscious.

Before you give first aid to a child who is conscious, tell the child who you are, and that you have training in first aid. If the child's parent or guardian is present, ask for permission to help the child. If present, the parent or legal guardian of a conscious or unconscious victim under the age of 18 should give consent before you give first aid.

If a child or infant is conscious but requires immediate emergency treatment, and a parent or guardian is not present, you do not need to wait for permission to help the child. The same is true if the child is unconscious. As with an adult, consent to give first aid is presumed. *Note:* The above advice is based on general principles of law. If you are interested in becoming informed about specific laws where you live, consult an attorney who is qualified to give legal advice in your state or jurisdiction.

Review Questions

Fill in the blanks with the right word or check the best answers.

3. Complete this list of four questions that you should ask when you first survey the scene in an emergency.
   a. Is the area _Safe_ for you and the victim?
   b. What actually _happened_ to the victim?
   c. How many people are _injured_ ?
   d. Are there any _people_ who can help?

4. Why should you identify yourself as a trained rescuer to the victim, parent or guardian, and bystanders?
   (Check **two**.)
   ☒ a. To comfort the victim
   ☒ b. So that someone already caring for the victim will know you are trained in first aid
   ☐ c. To learn the names of witnesses

Answers

3. When you first survey the scene in an emergency, you should ask these four questions:
   a. Is the area **safe** for you and the victim?
   b. What actually **happened** to the victim?
   c. How many people are **injured?**
   d. Are there any **bystanders** who can help?

4. You should identify yourself as a trained rescuer to the victim, parent or guardian, and bystanders—
   a. **To comfort the victim,** and
   b. **So that someone already caring for the victim will know you are trained in first aid.**

When you reach the injured person, you must find out what is wrong. An adult victim may be able to give you some information, but may not know about all of his or her injuries. It may be clear to you that a bone is broken or that there is bleeding, but there may be a more serious injury that you can't see. The pain from one injury may hide another injury.

If the victim is an infant or a child, the information you need will probably have to come from others. Even if the child can talk, he or she may not be able to explain what happened. Ask bystanders if they saw what happened.

Because an injured child or infant is usually frightened, it is very important for you to stay calm. Strangers who give first aid should try not to upset the child or infant even more. When you talk to the child or infant, speak simply and quietly. Say something like, "Hi, my name is _____, and I'm going to help you."

It is most helpful if a parent is nearby because—
1. The parent is usually the best person to calm the infant or child.
2. The parent will know about any medical problems.
3. You need the parent's consent, if the parent is present, before you begin to care for a conscious child or infant.

No matter what the emergency, follow the same basic steps to find out what is wrong with the victim. First, do a primary survey. Next, phone the EMS system for help. Then, do a secondary survey.

Do a Primary Survey

The primary survey is a series of checks to find conditions that are an immediate threat to a victim's life. When you do a primary survey, you are checking the condition of the body's two most important systems—the respiratory (breathing) system and the circulatory (blood flow) system. To do a primary survey, check the ABCs—

A—Airway: Does the person have an open airway (air passage that allows the person to breathe)?

B—Breathing: Is the person breathing?

C—Circulation: Is the person's heart beating? (Does the person have a pulse?) Is the person bleeding severely?

Note: "Severe bleeding" is bleeding that spurts from a wound with every beat of the heart. This is the only bleeding that must be controlled **immediately.** The rescuer should check for a pulse, then control any severe bleeding. You can learn how to control severe bleeding and other lifesaving skills in American Red Cross first aid courses.

If you find a problem with the person's **a**irway, **b**reathing or **c**irculation during a primary survey, then you must take care of it right away. In Chapter 2, you will find out how to open an adult's airway and check for breathing and circulation. You will find out how to do the same skills for children and infants in Chapters 7 and 10.

Review Questions

Check the best answer or fill in the blanks with the right letters.

5. The purpose of a primary survey is to—
   - ☑ a. Find conditions that are an immediate threat to life.
   - ☐ b. Find out if the person has any broken bones.

6. When you are doing a primary survey, you should check the person's **ABCs**:
   A _Airway_
   B _Breathing_
   C _Circulation_

Answers

5. **a.** The purpose of a primary survey is to **find conditions that are an immediate threat to life.**

6. When you are doing a primary survey, you should check the person's **ABC**s:
   A i r w a y
   B r e a t h i n g
   C i r c u l a t i o n (Check for pulse and severe bleeding.)

Phone the Emergency Medical Services (EMS) System for Help

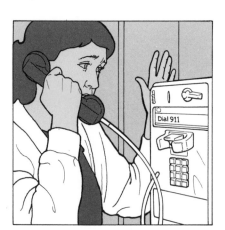

**Figure 2
Phone the EMS System**

After you have done a primary survey, you will have enough information about the victim's condition to give when you phone the EMS system. Depending on the situation, either you or a bystander should make the telephone call for help. Since you will be trained to deal with emergencies, it is usually best that you stay with the victim and send a bystander to phone the EMS system for help *(Fig. 2).* When you tell someone to call the EMS system, you should do the following:

1. Send two or more bystanders to make the call, if possible. This will make it more likely that the call is made.

2. Give the caller(s) the EMS telephone number to call. This number is 911 in some communities. Tell the caller(s) to dial "0" (the Operator) only if you do not know the special EMS number. Sometimes the emergency number is on the inside front cover of telephone directories and on pay phones.

3. Tell the caller(s) to give the dispatcher the following important facts:
   • **Where the emergency is located.** Give the exact address or location and the name of the city or town. It is helpful to give the names of nearby intersecting streets (cross streets), landmarks, the name of the building, the floor, and the room number.
   • **Telephone number from which the call is being made.**
   • **Caller's name.**
   • **What happened**—heart attack, cardiac arrest, car accident, house on fire, etc.
   • **How many people are injured.**
   • **Condition of the victim(s).**
   • **Help (first aid) being given.**

4. Tell the caller(s) not to hang up until the dispatcher hangs up. It is important to make sure the dispatcher has all the information needed to quickly send the right help to the scene.

5. Tell the caller(s) to report back to you after making the call and tell you what the dispatcher said.

Do a Secondary Survey

A secondary survey of the victim is a series of checks for injuries or other problems that are not an immediate threat to the victim's life, but that could cause problems later if they are not corrected. For example, during a secondary survey, the rescuer may find out that the person has a broken bone. This broken bone may not be immediately life threatening, but it could become a serious problem if ignored. A secondary survey has three steps:

1. Interview the victim. (Interview the parents or bystanders if the victim is unable to give you the necessary information.)
2. Determine if the victim's breathing, pulse, and body temperature *Vital signs* are normal.
3. Check the victim from head to toe, looking for injuries.

Most of the emergencies that you will learn about in this course will be discovered when you do a primary survey of the victim. For this reason, the secondary survey is not covered in detail in this course. However, you should interview a conscious heart attack victim as part of a secondary survey after you have sent someone to phone the EMS system for help. (The secondary survey is covered in detail in American Red Cross first aid courses.)

Interview the Victim

If the victim is conscious, talk to the victim to find out as much as you can. Reassure the victim that you can help him or her. Try to get his or her name and age; find out what happened. Does the person have any medical problems that might have led to this emergency? Ask if there is any pain, where it hurts, and for how long it has hurt. If the victim is unconscious, some of this information may be obtained from bystanders who know the victim or saw the accident.

This information is important for EMS and hospital emergency department personnel who will continue caring for the victim. It is important that you interview the victim and get this information as soon as possible because he or she may lose consciousness. Writing the information down will help you give it to EMS personnel accurately.

Review Questions

Check the best answer or fill in the blanks with the right word.

7. What is the chief purpose of a secondary survey?
   - ☒ a. To look for injuries or other problems that are not an immediate threat to life but that could be dangerous if not corrected
   - ☐ b. To find out the name of the victim's physician
   - ☐ c. To find out where the victim lives

8. When you phone for help, what should you tell the EMS dispatcher?
   - a. _Where_ the emergency is located.
   - b. _Phone_ _number_ from which the call is being made.
   - c. Your _name_.
   - d. What _happened_.
   - e. How many _injured_.
   - f. _Condition_ of victim(s).
   - g. _First aid_ being given.

9. Why is it important to interview a conscious heart attack victim?

☐ a. To be able to contact the victim's family and inform them fully about the victim's condition

☒ b. To get accurate information about the victim to give to EMS and emergency department personnel who will be caring for the victim

Answers

7. **a.** The chief purpose of a secondary survey is **to look for injuries or other problems that are not an immediate threat to life but that could be dangerous if not corrected.**

8. When you phone for help, you should tell the EMS dispatcher—
   a. **Where** the emergency is located.
   b. **Telephone number** from which the call is being made.
   c. Your **name.**
   d. What **happened.**
   e. How many **injured.**
   f. **Condition** of victim(s).
   g. **Help (first aid)** being given.

9. **b.** It is important to interview a conscious heart attack victim **to get accurate information about the victim to give to EMS and emergency department personnel who will be caring for the victim.**

Summary of Emergency Action Principles

Remember to follow these steps for all victims:
1. Survey the scene.
2. Do a primary survey.
3. Phone the EMS system for help.
4. Do a secondary survey.

If you find a problem during a primary survey, deal with it right away. For example, if the victim's heart has stopped, begin CPR and have someone phone the EMS system for help. In this case, you would not do a secondary survey. On the other hand, if you don't find any life-threatening problems during a primary survey, do a secondary survey. For example, if an adult victim is having a heart attack and is conscious, you should phone the EMS system for help and begin a secondary survey by interviewing the victim.

It is important for you and your community's EMS system to work together in an emergency. To learn more about your responsibilities as a rescuer and how your EMS system responds to a call for help, read the appendix, "The Emergency Medical Services (EMS) System," on page 291 of this workbook.

To help you prepare for an emergency, you should fill out the sheet, "Instructions for Emergency Phone Calls," at the end of this workbook. Post these instructions near a telephone in your home.

Unit One: Lifesaving Skills to Help Adults

How Much Do You Know About Heart Attacks and CPR?

Here are some questions about respiratory and cardiac emergencies in adults. These questions should help you think about your role in dealing with and preventing the types of emergencies covered in this class. **Check the best answers.** Do not feel disappointed if you are not able to answer every question correctly.

1. When someone has a heart attack, people often think of the attack as a sudden event. Later in this course, you will learn that most heart attacks are caused by a disease. At what age do you think the **disease** that causes heart attacks begins?
   - ☐ Heart disease begins around the age of 30.
   - ☒ Heart disease can begin in early childhood.

2. If you want to reduce your risk of having a heart attack, how can you do it?
   - ☒ You can reduce your risk of having a heart attack by having your blood pressure checked regularly, giving up smoking, and watching what you eat.
   - ☐ There is no way to reduce your risk of a heart attack.

3. Which of the following is a common signal of a heart attack?
   - ☒ A person having a heart attack may have pain or pressure in the chest.
   - ☐ A person having a heart attack may complain of pain in the legs.

4. What does CPR do?
   - ☐ CPR restarts the heart of a heart attack victim.
   - ☒ CPR supplies oxygen to the body's cells when a person's heart has stopped beating.

5. You arrive for work in the morning and find one of your friends lying on the floor. He is motionless and lying on his back. You kneel down, tap him on the shoulder, and ask him if he's OK. He doesn't answer you. You shout for help. What do you think a trained person would do next?
   - ☒ Check to see if the person is breathing and has a pulse.
   - ☐ Check for a medical ID bracelet that would tell what might be wrong.

6. What should you do for someone who is coughing hard and seems to have something caught in the throat?
   - ☒ Stay with the person, but do not interfere with the person's attempts to cough up the object.
   - ☐ Offer a glass of water, and instruct the person to drink it slowly.

Answers

1. **Heart disease can begin in early childhood.**
   Scientists think that cardiovascular disease, the disease that causes heart attacks, begins early in life, perhaps in early childhood. Studies have shown that some 19-year-olds already have partially clogged arteries that could cause heart attacks later in life.

2. **You can reduce your risk of having a heart attack by having your blood pressure checked regularly, giving up smoking, and watching what you eat.**
   These are three good ways of lowering your risk of having a heart attack, but there are more. In this course you will learn what causes heart attacks and what can be done to reduce the risk of dying from a heart attack.

3. **A person having a heart attack may have pain or pressure in the chest.**
   The most significant signal of a heart attack is pain and/or pressure in the chest. Other signals of a heart attack include sweating, nausea, and shortness of breath. Heart attack victims often try to deny the fact that they are having a heart attack. For this reason, being able to recognize that a person is having a heart attack is one very important skill that you will learn in this course. If you recognize a heart attack early, the victim's chances of surviving can be greatly improved.

4. **CPR supplies oxygen to the body's cells when a person's heart has stopped beating.**

   CPR is a way of supplying oxygen to the body's cells when a person's heart has stopped (cardiac arrest). It works because as you breathe air into the victim's lungs, oxygen enters the blood. Then, when you press on the chest, you move oxygen-carrying blood through the body. While many people think that CPR alone can save a victim of cardiac arrest by restarting the heart, it is really more complicated than that. CPR is used to keep the cells of the victim's body from dying until more advanced medical help arrives. It takes immediate CPR combined with the delivery of advanced emergency medical care within a short time, generally within 10 minutes, to give the victim the best chance of survival. Studies have shown that when CPR is combined with advanced emergency medical care, about 40 percent of the victims of cardiac arrest can be saved.

5. **Check to see if the person is breathing and has a pulse.**

   You must check the victim for the most serious problems first, and deal with these problems immediately to increase the victim's chances of survival. In an emergency situation, you should always follow the emergency action principles described in Chapter 1.

6. **Stay with the person, but do not interfere with the person's attempts to cough up the object.**

   If the person is coughing hard, he or she is also breathing. In that case, you should let the person try to cough up the object. In this course, you will learn how to tell if a person who is choking needs your help and what to do to clear the airway.

In this unit you will learn what to do for heart attacks and what you can do to prevent heart attacks from happening. You will learn how to begin care for an adult cardiac arrest victim by performing CPR. You will also learn how to give first aid to an adult who is choking or having some other breathing emergency that could lead to cardiac arrest.

Objectives

By the time you finish this section, you should be able to do the following:

1. Name the three leading causes of death for adults in the United States.

2. Explain how to reduce the chance of death from a heart attack.

3. Explain the purpose of CPR.

4. Describe what is needed to save the life of a victim of cardiac arrest.

5. Describe the citizen's role as a part of the emergency medical services (EMS) system.

What Unit One Will Teach You

You are visiting your cousin, David, and his wife, Ann. The three of you have just finished eating and are sitting in the backyard. After a few minutes, David stops talking.

"Are you feeling all right?" Ann asks.

"Sure, I'm OK," David says.

"Well, you don't look very OK to me," Ann replies.

"I had a little indigestion just before we ate, and I took something for it," he explains, "but it doesn't seem to be doing much good."

David is having a heart attack. His heart muscle is dying, making it difficult and painful for his heart to pump blood.

A moment later, David collapses. He is not breathing, and his heart has stopped beating—he is in **cardiac arrest.** Someone must help David immediately.

Two things must happen for David to have the best chance to live. CPR must be started right away, and advanced emergency medical care must get to David within 10 minutes.

David may be lucky if there is a CPR-trained bystander and his community has ambulances staffed with personnel trained to give advanced care. If David does not get prompt CPR and advanced emergency medical care, it is unlikely that he will survive.

Heart Disease Is the Number-One Killer

Cardiovascular disease, disease of the heart and blood vessels, is the leading cause of death for adults in the United States. Cancer is the second leading cause of death. The third leading cause of death is injury, of which automobile-related injuries are the most common **(Fig. 3).**

Overall, one in every five adult Americans has some form of cardiovascular disease. Or, put another way, one out of every five participants in this class is likely to have cardiovascular disease.

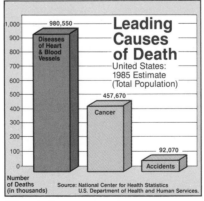

Figure 3
Leading Causes of Death

Reducing Deaths From Heart Attacks

Most people who die of a heart attack die before they ever reach a hospital. The best way to reduce deaths from heart attacks and cardiovascular disease is not simply to equip every hospital with the latest equipment and trained specialists, but to try to prevent the disease that causes heart attacks.

Many people believe that a heart attack occurs suddenly and by chance. This is rarely true. The disease that most often causes heart attacks (cardiovascular disease) is believed to begin in early childhood. The disease gets worse as a person gets older. As it gets worse, the chance of having a heart attack increases.

Preventing cardiovascular disease involves knowing what risk factors increase your chances of having a heart attack and knowing what you can do to control these risk factors.

Preventing death when a heart attack does occur involves recognizing the signals of a heart attack and knowing what to do. These topics will be discussed in more detail later in this course.

Most people who die of a heart attack die within two hours of the time when the heart attack signals start. Some victims die before anyone recognizes the need for emergency medical care. To save the lives of heart attack victims, emergency care must be immediately available in the community when a heart attack happens. This emergency care depends on citizens who are able to recognize the signals of a heart attack, provide first aid, and call for emergency medical services. Your being able to recognize the signals of a heart attack and acting quickly before the heart stops can mean the difference between life and death for many victims.

But if a person's heart has stopped (cardiac arrest), CPR is needed to keep oxygen-carrying blood flowing from the lungs to the brain and heart until more advanced emergency medical care arrives. The bystander who is able to give that lifesaving care could be you. Some experts estimate that if all victims of cardiac arrest received prompt CPR, followed by advanced emergency medical care within 10 minutes, many victims could be saved *(Fig. 4)*.

There are other situations, in addition to heart attacks, that can lead to cardiac arrest and the need for CPR. For example, victims of near-drowning, electric shock, drug overdose, and poisoning may go into cardiac arrest. If a person's heart stops for any reason, CPR must be started immediately, and advanced medical help must arrive within 10 minutes. You should also know that sometimes the heart just stops without warning.

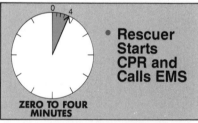

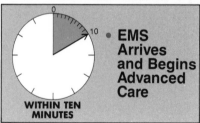

Figure 4
Critical Times for Saving a Life

Your Role

Rescuers—citizens like you—play a vital role both in preventing heart attacks from happening and in giving first aid when they do happen. When a cardiac or respiratory emergency occurs, it is up to you to recognize that emergency medical help is needed, to begin first aid, and to call your community's emergency medical services (EMS) system. Should cardiac arrest occur, you can use CPR to keep the brain and body cells supplied with oxygen during the critical minutes before the victim receives advanced emergency medical care.

Now let's return for a moment to the example given at the beginning of this section. If you had been trained in first aid, what could you have done to save David's life?

After David collapsed, you could have checked for breathing and pulse. You could have started CPR while telling someone to phone for emergency medical help. You could have continued to give CPR until David received advanced emergency medical care.

But there is something even more effective that you, as a trained rescuer, might have done. By recognizing the signals of a heart attack, you might have realized during dinner that something was seriously wrong with David. You then could have started first aid and called your community's EMS system for help. David might have received advanced emergency medical care before his heart stopped beating.

Review Questions

Fill in the blanks with the right word or check the best answer.

1. List the three leading causes of death for adults in the United States.
   a. _Cardiovascular desease_
   b. _Cancer_
   c. _Injuries_

2. When does the disease that causes heart attacks begin?
   ☐ a. Cardiovascular disease usually begins around the age of 50.
   ☐ b. Cardiovascular disease begins around the age of 30.
   ☑ c. Cardiovascular disease can begin in early childhood.

3. Assuming that CPR is started immediately after cardiac arrest, how soon must a victim receive advanced emergency medical care to have the best chance of survival?
   ☑ a. Within 10 minutes.
   ☐ b. Within 30 minutes.
   ☐ c. Within an hour.

Answers

1. The three leading causes of death for adults in the United States are—
   a. **Cardiovascular disease.**
   b. **Cancer.**
   c. **Injuries.**

2. c. **Cardiovascular disease can begin in early childhood.**

3. a. A victim of cardiac arrest must receive advanced emergency medical care **within 10 minutes** to have the best chance of survival.

2 What to Do When an Adult's Breathing Stops (Rescue Breathing)

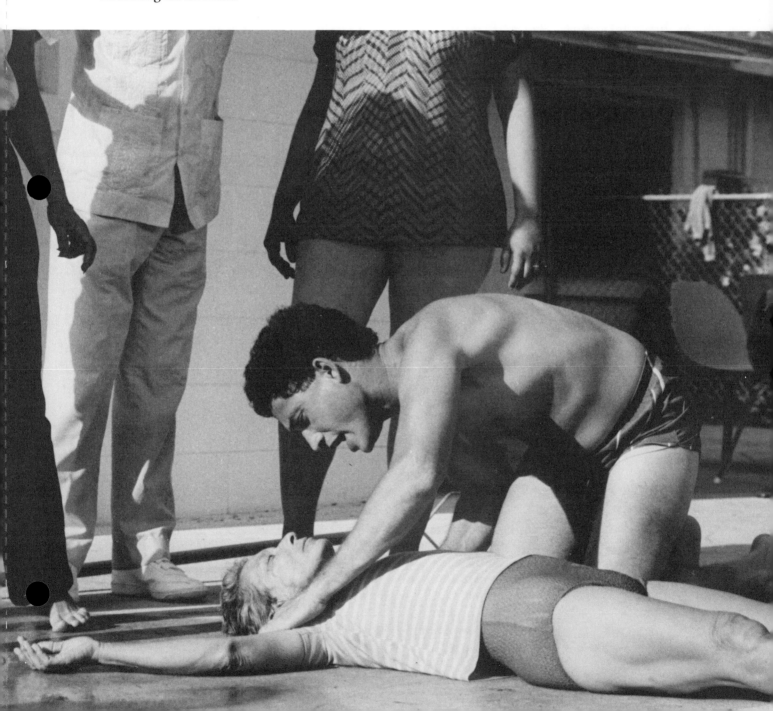

What to Do When an Adult's Breathing Stops (Rescue Breathing)

*In this chapter, you will learn how to give **artificial respiration**, also called **rescue breathing**. Rescue breathing is given to someone whose breathing has stopped but whose heart is still beating. A primary survey will tell you if you need to give rescue breathing.*

*You will also learn how respiratory emergencies happen, the purpose of rescue breathing, and why it works. You will practice checking the **ABCs** (Airway, Breathing, Circulation) when you do a primary survey, and you will also practice rescue breathing. You will practice some of these skills on each other and some on a manikin.*

Objectives

By the time you finish reading this chapter, you should be able to do the following:

1. *Describe how the respiratory and circulatory systems work to provide the body's cells with oxygen.*
2. *Describe the purpose of rescue breathing and how rescue breathing works.*
3. *Give one example of each of the two types of airway obstruction.*
4. *Describe when rescue breathing is needed.*
5. *Describe how to position a person for rescue breathing.*
6. *Describe how to give rescue breathing.*

Staying Alive

Your body is built from many millions of cells. To stay alive, these cells need a constant supply of oxygen. Right this minute, the vital flow of oxygen to your cells is being provided by two important body systems working together: the **respiratory system** and the **circulatory system.**

The **respiratory system** brings the oxygen needed to keep us alive into the body. Oxygen is part of the air we breathe. When we breathe in, air enters the body through the nose and mouth. It travels down the throat, through the windpipe, and into the lungs. The pathway from the nose and mouth to the lungs is called the **airway.** In order for air to enter the lungs, the airway must be open. In the lungs, the oxygen in the air is picked up by the blood and carried to all the cells of the body through the **circulatory system.**

If either the respiratory or circulatory system stops working or becomes damaged, then the supply of oxygen to the cells is decreased and the person may soon die. In cases like this, the victim needs rescue breathing or CPR to stay alive until advanced medical help arrives.

Respiratory Emergencies

A **respiratory emergency** occurs when a person's normal breathing stops or when breathing is so reduced that the person can't breathe enough air to stay alive. Without a constant supply of oxygen, the brain will begin to die after 4 to 6 minutes. In such cases, rescue breathing is needed immediately if the person is to live. Rescue breathing is a way of breathing air into someone's lungs when natural breathing has stopped or a person can't breathe properly on his or her own.

Rescue breathing works because the air you breathe into the victim contains more than enough oxygen to keep that person alive. The air you take in with every breath contains about 21 percent oxygen, but your body uses only a small part of that. The air you breathe out of your own lungs and into the lungs of the victim contains about 16 percent oxygen. That is enough oxygen to keep someone alive.

Causes of Respiratory Emergencies

Respiratory emergencies most commonly happen when the airway becomes obstructed in some way. There are two types of airway obstruction: **anatomic obstruction** and **mechanical obstruction.**

Anatomic obstruction occurs when the tongue or tissues of the throat block a person's airway. This can happen in two ways:

• The airway can be blocked by the back of the tongue dropping down into the throat. This is the most common cause of airway obstruction and often occurs when an unconscious person is lying on his or her back *(Fig. 5)*.

- The airway can be blocked when tissues in the throat swell. Swelling can be caused by injuries such as a blow to the neck, or by burns, allergies, insect stings and bites, poisons, and certain diseases and illnesses.

Mechanical obstruction occurs when the airway is partly or completely blocked by—

- A solid object, such as a piece of food or a small toy.
- Fluids, including vomit, blood, mucus, or saliva.

There are several other and less common causes of respiratory emergencies. Among them are electric shock, near-drowning, shock, breathing toxic substances, injury to the chest or lungs, and the effects of certain drugs. Additional information about the causes of respiratory emergencies in children and infants is given in Unit Two of this workbook.

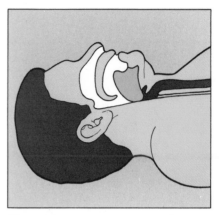

Figure 5
Tongue Obstructing Airway

Review Questions

Fill in the blanks with the right word or check the best answer.

1. You give rescue breathing when a person has stopped ___breathing___.

2. Rescue breathing works because the ___air___ you breathe out of your own lungs and into the lungs of the victim contains enough ___oxygen___ to keep the person alive until medical help arrives.

3. A person's airway can become obstructed if—
   a. The back of the ___tongue___ drops into the throat.
   b. The tissues in the ___throat___ swell.
   c. A ___solid___ ___object___ gets stuck in the airway.
   d. ___Fluids___ collect in the airway.

4. The most common cause of airway obstruction in an unconscious person is—
   ☒ a. The back of the tongue blocking the throat.
   ☐ b. An object blocking the airway.
   ☐ c. Fluids blocking the airway.

Answers

1. You give rescue breathing when a person has stopped **breathing**.

2. Rescue breathing works because the **air** you breathe out of your own lungs into the lungs of the victim contains enough **oxygen** to keep the person alive until medical help arrives.

3. A person's airway can become obstructed if—
   a. The back of the **tongue** drops into the throat.
   b. The tissues in the **throat** swell.
   c. A **solid object** gets stuck in the airway.
   d. **Fluids** collect in the airway.

4. a. The most common cause of airway obstruction in an unconscious person is **the back of the tongue blocking the throat**.

How to Give Rescue Breathing to an Adult

If you find someone collapsed on the floor, you should quickly survey the scene and do a primary survey.

1. **Check for Unresponsiveness**

   The first thing you should do is check to see if the person is conscious. Kneel down beside the person, tap or gently shake the person, and shout, "Are you OK?" *(Fig. 6)*.

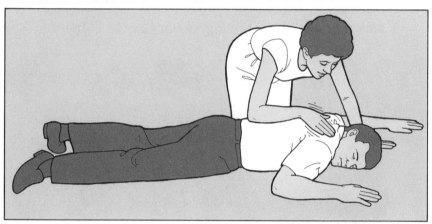

Figure 6
Check for Unresponsiveness

2. **Shout for Help**

   If the person does not move or answer, shout for help *(Fig. 7)*. You do this to get the attention of people you can ask to phone the EMS system for help after you complete a primary survey.

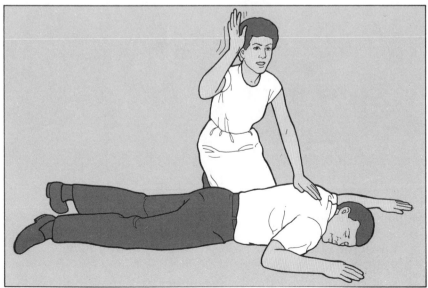

Figure 7
Shout for Help

No breathly but has a pulse

3. Position the Victim

Move the victim onto his or her back. To do this, roll the victim as a unit *(Fig. 8)*. This will help to avoid twisting the body and making any injuries worse. To position the victim—

- Kneel facing the victim, midway between the victim's hips and shoulders.
- Straighten the victim's legs, if necessary.
- Move the victim's arm closest to you so that it is stretched out above the victim's head.
- Lean over the victim and place one hand on the victim's shoulder and the other on the victim's hip.

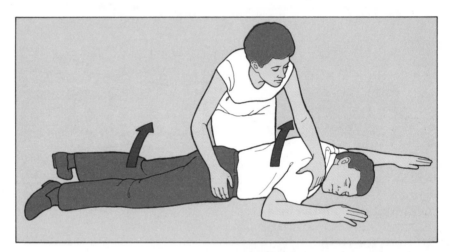

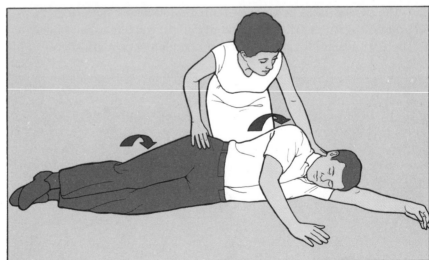

Figure 8
Position the Victim

- Roll the victim toward you as a single unit by pulling slowly and evenly.
- As you roll the victim onto his or her back, move your hand from the shoulder to support the back of the head and neck.

- Place the victim's arm closest to you alongside the victim's body.

It is important to position the victim on his or her back as quickly as possible. It should take no more than <u>10 seconds</u> to do this.

Note: Most conditions requiring rescue breathing or CPR are not due to or associated with major injuries. However, some victims who require rescue breathing or CPR may have received a serious injury to the head, neck, or back. Moving these victims or opening the airway as described below may result in further injury. Additional methods for handling these victims are discussed in the American Red Cross CPR: Basic Life Support for the Professional Rescuer course.

4. **"A"—Open the Airway**

Immediately open the victim's airway. This is the most important action for successful resuscitation. The technique for opening the airway is called the **head-tilt/chin-lift**. The head-tilt/chin-lift lifts the tongue away from the back of the throat and opens the airway. It is done by tilting the person's head back and, at the same time, lifting up on the chin *(Fig. 9)*. To open the airway—

- Place your hand—the one nearest the victim's head—on the victim's forehead and apply firm backward pressure with the palm of your hand to tilt the head back.
- Place the fingers of your other hand under the bony part of the victim's lower jaw near the chin and lift to bring the chin forward.
- Lift the jaw until the teeth are nearly brought together. Do not close the victim's mouth. You can use your thumb to help keep the mouth open. Do not press on the soft tissue under the chin. This might close the airway.

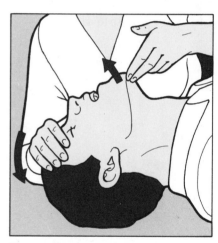

Figure 9
Head-Tilt/Chin-Lift

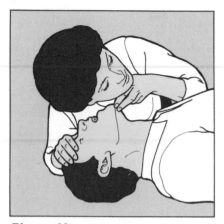

Figure 10
Check for Breathlessness

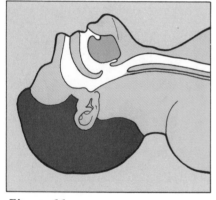

Figure 11
An Open Airway

5. **"B"—Check for Breathlessness** (Look, listen, and feel for breathing.)

With the head tilted back and the chin lifted, check to see if the victim is breathing *(Fig. 10)*. Tilting the head back opens the airway and may in itself restore breathing *(Fig. 11)*.

To check breathing—

- Keep the victim's head tilted back and the chin lifted to keep the airway open.
- Place your ear just above the victim's mouth and nose and look at the victim's chest.
- Look, listen, and feel. **Look** for the chest to rise and fall, **listen** for breathing, and **feel** for air coming out of the victim's nose and mouth. Do this for 3 to 5 seconds.

If the victim is breathing, you will see chest movement and hear and feel air escaping at your ear and cheek. Chest movement alone does not mean that the victim is breathing, so be sure to look, listen, and feel for breathing.

6. Give 2 Full Breaths

If the victim is not breathing, you must get air into his or her lungs at once *(Fig. 12).* To give breaths—

- While keeping the airway open with the head-tilt/chin-lift, gently pinch the victim's nose shut with the thumb and index finger of the hand that is maintaining backward pressure on the forehead.
- Open your mouth wide. Take a deep breath. Seal your lips tightly around the outside of the victim's mouth.
- Give 2 full breaths at the rate of 1 to 1½ seconds per breath. Pause between breaths just long enough for you to take another breath. Watch for the chest to rise while you breathe into the victim. Watch for the chest to fall after you remove your mouth from the victim. Listen and feel for air escaping as the victim's chest falls.

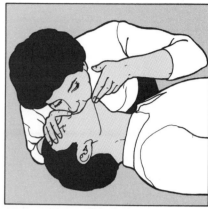

Figure 12
Mouth-to-Mouth Breathing

If you feel resistance when you breathe into the victim and air will not go in, the most likely cause is that you may not have tilted the head back far enough and the tongue may be blocking the airway. Retilt the head and give 2 full breaths. If air still does not go into the victim's lungs, the victim's airway may be blocked by food or some other material. Chapter 3 describes how to help an adult with an airway obstruction caused by food or another object.

7. "C"—Check Circulation by Checking for a Pulse at the Side of the Neck

Check to see if the victim's heart is beating by feeling for a pulse at the side of the neck. This pulse is called the **carotid pulse** *(Fig. 13).* To check for a carotid pulse—

- While keeping the victim's head tilted back with one hand on the forehead, use your other hand to find the pulse. First, place your index and middle fingers on the Adam's apple. (Everyone has an Adam's apple.) Then slide your fingers toward you into the groove between the windpipe and the muscle at the side of the neck. This is where the carotid pulse is located.
- Press gently with your fingertips to feel for the beat of the pulse. Be sure to feel for the pulse on the side of the neck closest to you. **Do not use your thumb** because you may feel your own pulse. Feel for the carotid pulse for 5 to 10 seconds.

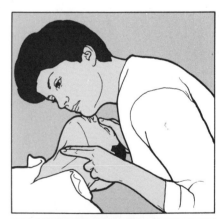

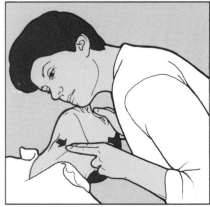

Figure 13
Locate and Feel Carotid Pulse

8. Phone the EMS System

After you have checked the pulse, you will have enough information about the victim's condition to give to the bystanders you are sending to phone the EMS system. In Chapter 1, you learned what to tell bystanders when calling the EMS system. Now you can add the last important piece of information: details of the victim's condition. Tell the bystanders whether the victim is conscious, breathing, and has a pulse. Tell them to give this information to the EMS dispatcher.

9. Begin Rescue Breathing

If you feel a pulse and the victim is not breathing, then begin rescue breathing. (If you do not feel a pulse, the victim's heart has stopped and you must start CPR, which you will learn in Chapter 5.) To give rescue breathing—

- Keep the airway open.
- Give 1 breath every 5 seconds. Each breath should last for 1 to 1½ seconds. A good way to time the breaths is to count, "One one-thousand, two one-thousand, three one-thousand, four one-thousand." Take a breath yourself, and then breathe into the victim. Watch for the chest to rise as you breathe into the victim.
- Between breaths, remove your mouth from the victim. Look for the chest to fall as you listen and feel at the victim's mouth and nose for escaping air. You should also listen to hear if the victim starts breathing again.

10. Recheck Pulse

After 1 minute of rescue breathing (about 12 breaths), you should check the victim's pulse. To check the pulse—

- Keep the airway open and feel for the carotid pulse for 5 seconds.

If there is a pulse, then check for breathing for 3 to 5 seconds. If the victim is breathing, keep the airway open and monitor breathing and pulse closely. This means that you should look, listen, and feel for breathing while you keep checking the pulse. If the victim is not breathing, continue rescue breathing and keep checking the pulse once every minute.

Continue to give rescue breathing (steps 9 and 10 above) until one of the following happens:

- The victim begins breathing on his or her own.
- Another trained rescuer takes over for you.
- EMS personnel arrive and take over.
- You are too exhausted to continue.

Review Questions

Fill in the blanks with the right word or check the best answer.

5. You see someone collapse on the sidewalk in front of you. You survey the scene and decide it is safe. What should you do upon reaching the victim?
Check for _breathing_, position the victim, if necessary, and open the _airway_.

6. How do you open the airway?
   - ☒ a. Tilt the head and lift the chin.
   - ☐ b. Blow into the victim's nose.
   - ☐ c. Push down on the chin.

7. How often should you give rescue breaths to an adult?
   - ☐ a. Give 1 breath every second.
   - ☒ b. Give 1 breath every 5 seconds.
   - ☐ c. Give 1 breath every 30 seconds.

8. You should continue rescue breathing until one of four things happens. These four things are—
   a. The victim starts _breathing_.
   b. _EMS_ _personnel_ arrive and take over.
   c. Another trained rescuer _takes_ _over_ for you.
   d. You are too _tired_ to continue.

Answers

5. If you see someone collapse, you should check for **unresponsiveness,** position the victim, if necessary, and open the **airway**.

6. a. To open the airway, **tilt the head and lift the chin.**

7. b. When giving rescue breaths to an adult, **give 1 breath every 5 seconds.**

8. You should continue rescue breathing until one of the following happens:
   a. The victim starts **breathing.**
   b. **EMS personnel** arrive and take over.
   c. Another trained rescuer **takes over** for you.
   d. You are too **exhausted** to continue.

More About Rescue Breathing for an Adult

Air in the Stomach

Sometimes during rescue breathing the rescuer may breathe air into the victim's stomach. Air in the stomach can be a serious problem. It can cause the victim to vomit. When an unconscious person vomits, the stomach contents may go into the lungs. That can lead to death.

Air can enter the stomach in three ways:

- When the rescuer keeps breathing into the victim after the chest has risen. This causes extra air to fill the stomach.
- When the rescuer has not tilted the victim's head back far enough to open the airway completely and must breathe at greater pressure to fill the victim's lungs.
- When the rescue breaths are given too quickly. Quick breaths are given with higher pressure, which causes air to enter the stomach.

To avoid forcing air into the stomach, make sure you keep the victim's head tilted all the way back. Breathe into the victim only enough to make the chest rise. Don't give breaths too quickly; pause between breaths long enough to let the victim's lungs empty and for you to take another breath yourself.

If you notice that the victim's stomach has begun to bulge, make sure that the head is tilted back far enough and make sure you are not breathing into the victim too hard and too fast.

Vomiting

Sometimes while you are helping an unconscious victim, the victim may vomit. If this happens, turn the victim's head and body to the side, quickly wipe the material out of the victim's mouth, and continue where you left off.

Mouth-to-Nose Breathing

There are a few situations in which you may not be able to make a good enough seal over a person's mouth to perform rescue breathing. For example, the person's jaw or mouth may have been injured during an accident, or the jaw may be shut too tight to open, or your mouth may be too small. In such cases, **mouth-to-nose breathing** should be done as follows:

- Maintain the backward head-tilt position with one hand on the forehead. Use the other hand to close the mouth *(Fig. 14),* making sure to push on the chin and not on the throat.
- Open your mouth wide, take a deep breath, seal your mouth tightly around the person's nose, and breathe full breaths into the person's nose *(Fig. 15),* as described in step 9 on page 38. Open the person's mouth between breaths, if possible, to allow air to come out *(Fig. 16).*

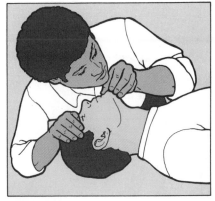

Figure 14
Close Mouth for Mouth-to-Nose Breathing

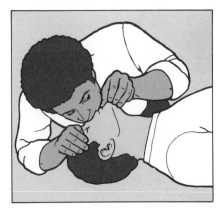

Figure 15
Mouth-to-Nose Breathing

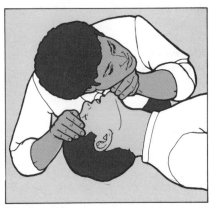

Figure 16
Check for Air Coming Out

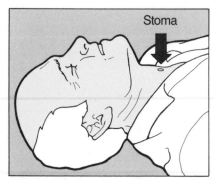

Figure 17
Victim With a Stoma

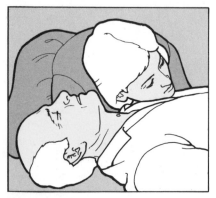

Figure 18
Check for Breathing

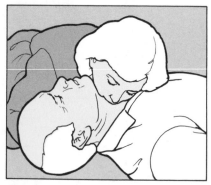

Figure 19
Mouth-to-Stoma Breathing

Mouth-to-Stoma Breathing

There are some people who have had surgery to remove all or part of the upper end of their windpipe. They breathe through an opening called a **stoma** in the front of the neck *(Fig. 17)*. This takes the air right into the windpipe, bypassing both the mouth and nose.

Most people with this condition wear a bracelet or necklace or carry a card identifying their condition. In an emergency, you may not have time to search for a medical card, so it is important to look at the neck area during the primary survey to see if the person has a stoma.

To give rescue breathing to someone with a stoma, you must give breaths through the stoma and not through the mouth or nose.

In **mouth-to-stoma** breathing, you follow the same basic steps as in mouth-to-mouth breathing, except that you—

1. Look, listen, and feel for breathing with your ear held over the stoma *(Fig. 18)*.
2. Give breaths into the stoma, breathing at the same rate as for mouth-to-mouth breathing *(Fig. 19)*.

There are several other important things you should remember when you give rescue breathing to someone who breathes through a stoma:

- Don't tilt the victim's head back.
- Don't breathe air into the victim through his or her nose or mouth. This may fill the victim's stomach with air.
- Never block the stoma, since it is the only way the victim has to breathe.
- In some instances, a person who has had only part of the upper end of his or her windpipe removed may breathe through the stoma as well as the nose and mouth. If the person's chest does not rise when you breathe through the stoma, you should close off the mouth and nose *(Fig. 20)* and continue breathing through the stoma.

Victims with Dentures (False Teeth)

If a person who needs rescue breathing is wearing dentures, leave the dentures in place if they have not moved. They will give support to the mouth and cheeks during mouth-to-mouth breathing. Even if the dentures are loose, the head-tilt/chin-lift described earlier may help keep them in place. If the dentures become so loose that they block the airway or make it difficult for you to give breaths, take them out.

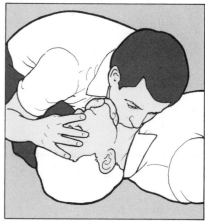

Figure 20
Mouth-to-Stoma Breathing for Partial Stoma

Practice Sessions: Information and Directions

Introduction

During this course, you will practice the skills that are demonstrated on video or film. There will be a practice session after each video or film. In the practice sessions you will learn how to do rescue breathing, how to help someone who is choking, and how to do CPR (cardiopulmonary resuscitation). You will learn these skills for adults, children, and infants.

During each practice session you will use a skill sheet to help you learn a particular skill. There are directions on the page before each skill sheet. Please read the directions carefully before you start each practice session.

Skill Sheet

The skill sheet contains step-by-step directions on how to perform each skill. There are also pictures to show you what to do. The left side of each page is used as a checklist. There are two columns of boxes. One column is labeled Partner Check; the other is labeled Instructor Check.

Most skill sheets have a section at the end called "What to Do Next." This section will help you decide on the correct first aid if a victim's condition changes.

How to Practice

You will practice each skill in groups of two or three people. You will practice most of the skills on a manikin, taking turns to practice.

One person will be the rescuer and will practice the skills. The second person will act as partner. The partner will read the directions on the skill sheet to the rescuer. If there are three people in your group, the third person will watch to see if the skills are done correctly. After the first rescuer has finished practicing, change places. Each person must practice on the manikin.

For some skills, you will practice on one another and not on a manikin. When you do this, you will take turns being the victim.

If you need help, ask your instructor.

Directions for the Rescuer

When you begin practice, have your partner read the skill sheet to you. Your partner should read each step as you practice so you will know what to do.

At some points in the practice, your partner will give you some information about the victim. This is to make the practice seem more like a real emergency. In a real emergency, you would discover this information as you gave first aid.

Practice until you can perform the skills correctly. **Practice** until you feel confident doing the skills. **Practice** until you can perform the skills in the right order, without any directions from your partner.

When you can do this, ask your partner to check you. As you do each step of the procedure, your partner should check the appropriate box in the Partner Check column on the skill sheet.

At the end of most skill sheets is a section called "What to Do Next." Your partner will read this section to you only after you are confident that you know the skill. This section will give you practice in deciding how to change the care you are giving in response to changes in the victim's condition. Your partner will give you information about the victim's condition, and you will decide what to do next.

Instructions for the Partner

You should read the directions on the skill sheet to the rescuer. When the rescuer can do the skills correctly without any coaching, begin the Partner Check. When you do the Partner Check, have the rescuer go through the procedure. As the rescuer demonstrates the skill, read the information wherever the skill sheet says, "Partner/ Instructor says. . . ." Do not give any other directions unless you see the rescuer doing something wrong. As the rescuer does each step correctly, check the box by that step in the Partner Check column.

When the rescuer can demonstrate the whole procedure correctly, read one of the statements in the "What to Do Next" section at the appropriate point in the procedure.

If the rescuer can't go through the whole procedure correctly, help the rescuer practice some more.

Instructor Skill Test

When all the members of your group have practiced and are ready to be tested, ask the instructor to test your skills. During the skill test, the instructor will ask you to go through the whole procedure without coaching. When you have completed the procedure correctly, the instructor will sign your workbook.

If the instructor sees a serious error, he or she will stop you and correct you. You will be asked to practice some more before being tested again. Ask your partner to work with you. When you have practiced and feel that you are ready to be tested again, ask the instructor to retest you.

Practice on Each Other

As stated above, you will practice some skills on a partner. By practicing on each other, you will learn how it feels to work on a real person. For example, you will learn how a real carotid pulse feels.

When practicing on a partner, follow the skill sheet directions but **do not make mouth-to-mouth contact; do not give actual rescue breaths; do not do chest compressions; and do not do abdominal thrusts or chest thrusts.**

Practice on a Manikin

Before you practice on the manikin, clean its face and the inside of its mouth. Directions for doing this are given in the section called "Some Health Precautions and Guidelines to Follow During This Course" on page 3 of this workbook. **Be sure that the manikin's face and mouth have been cleaned before each new member of your group practices, and whenever you change places and begin to practice on the manikin.**

Because it is important to keep the manikin's face clean, the manikin should always be lying on its back. Do not turn the manikin on its face or side to practice positioning the victim. Check for unresponsiveness; then go directly to the step, "Open the Airway."

Health Precautions

Before you start practicing, read "Some Health Precautions and Guidelines to Follow During This Course" on page 3 of this workbook. If you have any questions or if there is any reason that you should not take part in the practice sessions, it is important that you talk with your instructor.

Practice Session: Rescue Breathing for an Adult

The rescue breathing practice session is the first practice session in Unit One. During this practice session, you will first practice on a partner. If possible, a third person should read the skill sheet as you practice on a partner.

Remember: When you practice on a partner, **do not make mouth-to-mouth contact or give actual rescue breaths.**

Next you will practice on a manikin. When you practice on a manikin, you will practice all the steps and will give actual rescue breaths.

Before you start practicing, carefully read the skill sheet on pages 47 through 50. If you don't remember how to use the checklist, read pages 44 through 46.

Before you practice on the manikin, clean its face and the inside of its mouth. Directions for doing this are given in the section called "Some Health Precautions and Guidelines to Follow During This Course" on page 3 of this workbook. Clean the manikin's face and mouth before each person in your group practices.

Skill Sheet: Rescue Breathing for an Adult

You find a person lying on the ground, not moving. You should survey the scene to see if it is safe and to get some idea of what happened. Then do a primary survey by checking the ABCs.

Remember: When using a real person as a victim, **do not make mouth-to-mouth contact or give actual rescue breaths.**

Partner Check
Instructor Check

☐ ☐ **Check for Unresponsiveness**

Tap or gently shake victim.

Rescuer shouts, "Are you OK?"

Partner/Instructor says, "Unconscious."

Rescuer repeats, "Unconscious."

Rescuer shouts, "Help!"

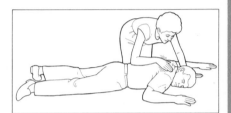

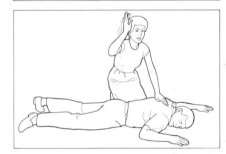

Position the Victim

Roll victim onto back, if necessary.

Kneel facing victim, midway between victim's hips and shoulders.

Straighten victim's legs, if necessary, and move victim's arm closest to you above victim's head.

Lean over victim, and place one hand on victim's shoulder and other hand on victim's hip.

Roll victim toward you as a single unit. As you roll victim, move your hand from victim's shoulder to support back of head and neck.

Place victim's arm closest to you alongside victim's body.

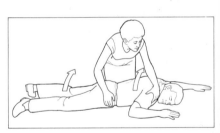

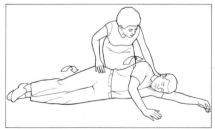

Partner Check
Instructor Check

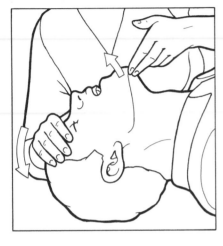

☐ ☐ **Open the Airway** (Use head-tilt/chin-lift)

Place your hand—the one nearest the victim's head—on the victim's forehead.

Place fingers of other hand under bony part of lower jaw near chin.

Tilt head and lift jaw. Avoid closing victim's mouth. Avoid pushing on the soft parts under the chin.

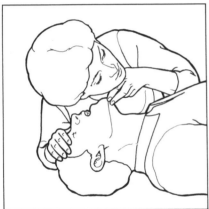

☐ ☐ **Check for Breathlessness**

Maintain open airway with head-tilt/chin-lift.

Place your ear over victim's mouth and nose.

Look at chest; listen and feel for breathing for 3 to 5 seconds.

Partner/Instructor says, "No breathing."

Rescuer repeats, "No breathing."

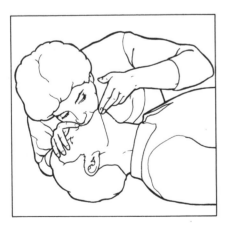

☐ ☐ **Give 2 Full Breaths**

Maintain open airway with head-tilt/chin-lift.

Pinch nose shut.

Open your mouth wide, take a deep breath, and seal your lips tightly around outside of victim's mouth.

Give 2 full breaths at the rate of 1 to 1½ seconds per breath. Pause between each breath for you to take a breath.

Look for the chest to rise and fall; listen and feel for escaping air.

Partner Check
Instructor Check

☐ ☐ **Check for Pulse**

Maintain head-tilt with one hand on forehead.

Locate Adam's apple with middle and index fingers of hand nearest victim's feet.

Slide fingers down into groove of neck on side closest to you.

Feel for carotid pulse for 5 to 10 seconds.

Partner/Instructor says, "No breathing, but there is a pulse."

Rescuer repeats, "No breathing, but there is a pulse."

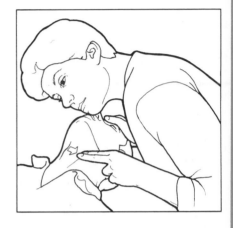

☐ ☐ **Phone the EMS System for Help**

Tell someone to call for an ambulance.

Rescuer says, "No breathing, has a pulse, call _____."
(*Local emergency number or Operator*)

☐ ☐ **Now Begin Rescue Breathing**

Maintain open airway with head-tilt/chin-lift.

Pinch nose shut.

Open your mouth wide, take a deep breath, and seal your lips tightly around outside of victim's mouth.

Give 1 breath every 5 seconds at the rate of 1 to 1½ seconds per breath. Count aloud, "One one-thousand, two one-thousand, three one-thousand, four one-thousand." Take a breath yourself, and then breathe into the victim.

Look for the chest to rise and fall; listen and feel for escaping air and the return of breathing.
Continue for 1 minute—about 12 breaths.

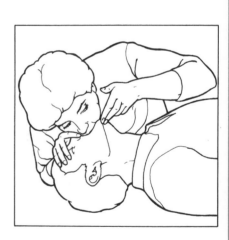

Practice Session: Rescue Breathing for an Adult

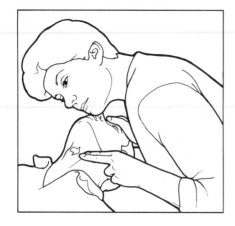

Partner Check
Instructor Check

☐ ☑ **Recheck Pulse**

Maintain head-tilt with one hand on forehead.

Locate carotid pulse and feel for 5 seconds.

Partner/Instructor says, "Has a pulse."

Rescuer repeats, "Has a pulse."

Look, listen, and feel for breathing for 3 to 5 seconds.

Partner/Instructor says, "No breathing."

Rescuer repeats, "No breathing."

☐ ☑ **Continue Rescue Breathing**

Maintain open airway with head-tilt/chin-lift.

Give 1 breath every 5 seconds at the rate of 1 to 1½ seconds per breath.

Recheck pulse every minute.

☐ ☑ **What to Do Next**

While the rescuer is rechecking pulse and breathing, the partner should read one of the following statements:

1. Victim is breathing but is still unconscious.

2. Victim has a pulse but is not breathing.

Based on this information, the rescuer should decide what to do next and continue giving the right care.

Final Instructor Check _M.E.A_

50

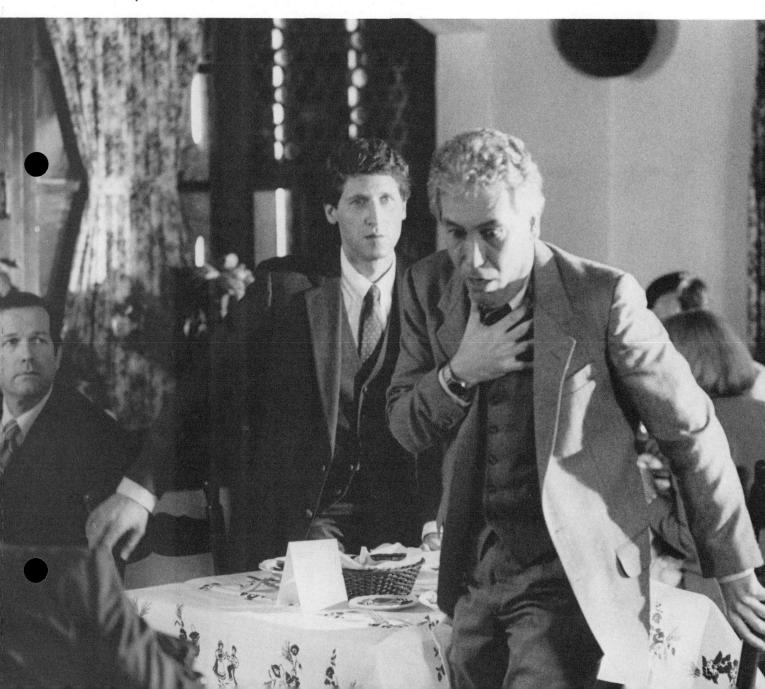

When someone's airway gets blocked by a piece of food or some other object, the person can quickly stop breathing, lose consciousness, and die. In this chapter, you will learn how to tell if an adult is choking (has an airway obstruction). You will learn how to tell whether the person has an airway obstruction that requires first aid, and you will learn the first aid to clear an obstructed airway.

Objectives

By the time you finish this chapter, you should be able to do the following:

1. *List at least two reasons why people choke.*
2. *Describe the difference between airway obstructions that require first aid and those obstructions that can best be cleared by the victim's own efforts.*
3. *Describe the first aid for a conscious victim who is choking.*
4. *Describe the first aid for an unconscious victim who is choking.*

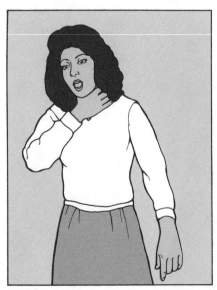

Figure 21
Universal Distress Signal for Choking

Causes and Signals of Choking

About 3,000 people will choke to death this year. Here are the most common actions that lead to choking:

- Trying to swallow large pieces of food that are poorly chewed.
- Drinking alcohol before or during eating. Alcohol dulls the nerves that help you swallow.
- Wearing dentures (false teeth). Dentures make it difficult to sense the size of food when chewing and swallowing.
- Eating while talking excitedly or laughing, or eating too fast.
- Walking, playing, or running with objects in the mouth.

Choking is sometimes mistaken for a heart attack or other serious condition. When this happens, the right kind of care may be delayed or the wrong kind of care may be given, so it is important to know how to recognize when someone is choking.

Being able to recognize an airway obstruction is the key to saving the victim. There are two types of obstruction that you need to know about—**partial airway obstruction** and **complete airway obstruction.** It is important to be able to recognize the difference between the two.

Partial Airway Obstruction

With partial airway obstruction, the person may have either good air exchange or poor air exchange.

- When a person has **partial airway obstruction with good air exchange,** he or she can cough forcefully. He or she may also wheeze between breaths. **If the person is able to cough forcefully on his or her own, do not interfere with attempts to cough up the object**. You should stay with the person and encourage him or her to continue coughing. If coughing persists, call the EMS system for help.
- When a person has **partial airway obstruction with poor air exchange,** he or she will have a weak, ineffective cough and may make a high-pitched noise while breathing. An obstruction may begin with poor air exchange, or it may begin with good air exchange and turn into an obstruction with poor air exchange. **Partial airway obstruction with poor air exchange should be dealt with as if it were complete airway obstruction.**

Complete Airway Obstruction

When there is complete obstruction of the airway, the person will not be able to speak, breathe, or cough. The person may clutch at his or her throat with one or both hands. This is the universal distress signal for choking *(Fig. 21)*. You must act right away to clear the airway.

Review Questions

Fill in the blanks with the right word or check the best answer.

1. These common actions can lead to choking—
   a. Trying to swallow poorly chewed _chewed_ .
   b. Drinking _alcohol_ before and during eating.
   c. Wearing _dentures_ , which make it difficult to sense the size of food.
   d. Eating while talking excitedly or laughing, or _eating_ too fast.
   e. Walking, playing, or running with objects in the _mouth_ .

2. A choking victim is coughing forcefully. You should—
   ☐ a. Slap the person on the back.
   ☒ b. Stay with the person and encourage him or her to continue coughing.
   ☐ c. Perform abdominal thrusts.

3. A person is coughing weakly and having great difficulty breathing. You should—
   ☒ a. Give first aid for complete airway obstruction.
   ☐ b. Leave the person alone and watch him or her.

4. What is the universal distress signal for choking?
   ☒ a. Clutching at the throat
   ☐ b. Coughing forcefully
   ☐ c. High-pitched wheezing

Answers

1. These common actions can lead to choking—
   a. Trying to swallow poorly chewed **food.**
   b. Drinking **alcohol** before and during eating.
   c. Wearing **dentures** (false teeth), which make it difficult to sense the size of food.
   d. Eating while talking excitedly or laughing, or **eating** too fast.
   e. Walking, playing, or running with objects in the **mouth**.

2. b. When a choking victim is coughing forcefully, you should **stay with the person and encourage him or her to continue coughing.**

3. a. If a person is coughing weakly and having great difficulty breathing, you should **give first aid for complete airway obstruction.**

4. a. The universal distress signal for choking is **clutching at the throat.**

First Aid for a Conscious Adult With a Complete Airway Obstruction

If you see someone who seems to be choking, survey the scene as you approach the victim.

1. Begin a primary survey by asking, "Are you choking?" If the person is coughing weakly or making high-pitched noises or is not able to speak, breathe, or cough forcefully, tell the person that you are trained in first aid and offer to help.
2. If you are alone, shout for help. If there is a bystander, have that person phone the EMS system for help.
3. Do abdominal thrusts (sometimes called the Heimlich maneuver) as follows:
    *   Stand behind the victim. The victim may be either standing or sitting. Wrap your arms around his or her waist. Make a fist with one hand. Place the thumb side of your fist against the middle of the victim's abdomen, just above the navel and well below the lower tip of the breastbone *(Figs. 22, 23, and 24)*.

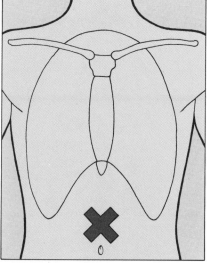

Figure 22
Location for Abdominal Thrusts

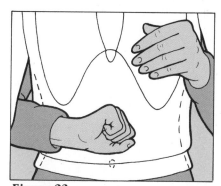

Figure 23
Location for Abdominal Thrusts

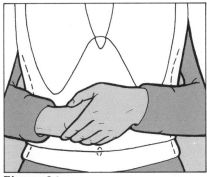

Figure 24
Hand Placement for Abdominal Thrusts

55

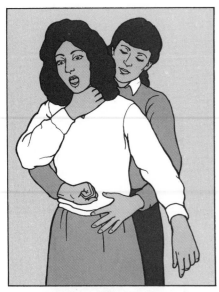

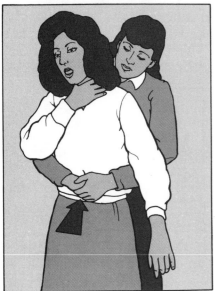

Figure 25
Giving Abdominal Thrusts

- Grasp your fist with your other hand. Keeping your elbows out from the victim, press your fist into the person's abdomen with a quick upward thrust *(Fig. 25)*. Be sure that your fist is directly on the midline of the victim's abdomen when you press. Do not direct the thrusts to the right or to the left. Think of each thrust as a separate and distinct attempt to dislodge the object.
- Repeat the thrusts until the obstruction is cleared or until the person becomes unconscious.

Later in this chapter, you will learn how to help a choking victim who becomes unconscious.

If You Are Alone and Choking

If you are choking and there is no one around to help, you can do an abdominal thrust on yourself. Make a fist with one hand and place the thumb side on the middle of your abdomen slightly above the navel and well below the tip of your breastbone. Grasp your fist with your other hand and give a quick upward thrust. You can also lean forward and press your abdomen over any firm object such as the back of a chair, a railing, or a sink. Be careful not to lean over anything with a sharp edge or corner that might injure you.

Review Questions

Check the best answer.

5. Abdominal thrusts are given to a victim who is—
   - ☒ a. Coughing weakly and making high-pitched noises.
   - ☐ b. Coughing forcefully and wheezing between breaths.

6. When you give abdominal thrusts, what part of your fist do you place against the victim?
   - ☐ a. The palm side
   - ☒ b. The thumb side
   - ☐ c. The knuckles

7. When you give abdominal thrusts, where do you place your fist?
   - ☐ a. At the lower tip of the breastbone
   - ☒ b. Just above the navel and well below the lower tip of the breastbone
   - ☐ c. On the navel

8. Abdominal thrusts are given—
   - ☒ a. With a quick upward thrust.
   - ☐ b. Straight back.
   - ☐ c. Inward and downward.

Answers

5. a. Abdominal thrusts are given to a victim who is **coughing weakly and making high-pitched noises.**

6. b. When you give abdominal thrusts, place **the thumb side** of your fist against the victim.

7. b. When you give abdominal thrusts, place your fist **just above the navel and well below the lower tip of the breastbone.**

8. a. Abdominal thrusts are given **with a quick upward thrust.**

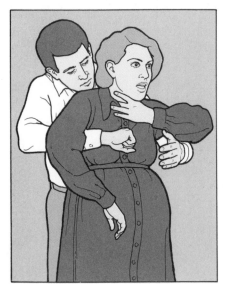

Figure 26
Hand Placement for Chest Thrusts

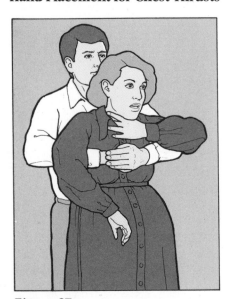

Figure 27
Giving Chest Thrusts

Chest Thrusts for a Conscious Adult

You may not be able to get your arms around the waist of some choking victims to deliver effective abdominal thrusts. For example, the person may be greatly overweight or in the late stages of pregnancy. In the case of a person who is in the late stages of pregnancy, abdominal thrusts could be dangerous. In both cases, chest thrusts are performed instead. Chest thrusts are done in the following way:

1. With the person either standing or sitting, stand behind the person and place your arms under the person's armpits and around the chest. Place the thumb side of your fist on the middle of the breastbone. Be sure that your fist is centered right on the breastbone and not on the ribs. Also make sure that your fist is not near the lower tip of the breastbone *(Fig. 26).*

2. Grasp your fist with your other hand and give backward thrusts *(Fig. 27).*

3. Give thrusts until the obstruction is cleared or until the person loses consciousness. You should think of each thrust as a separate and distinct attempt to dislodge the object.

When to Stop Thrusts

You should stop giving abdominal or chest thrusts immediately if the object is coughed up or the person begins to breathe or cough. Watch the person and make sure that the object has been removed from the airway and that the person is breathing freely again. Even after the object is coughed up, the person may have problems in breathing that are not clear to you. You should also realize that both abdominal thrusts and chest thrusts may cause internal injuries. Therefore, **the person should be taken to the nearest hospital emergency department even if he or she seems to be breathing without difficulty.**

Review Questions

Check the best answer.

9. If a choking victim is greatly overweight or in the late stages of pregnancy, you should give—
   - ☐ a. Abdominal thrusts.
   - ☒ b. Chest thrusts.

10. When giving chest thrusts, place your fist—
    - ☒ a. On the middle of the breastbone.
    - ☐ b. On the lower end of the breastbone.
    - ☐ c. On the navel.

11. You are giving chest thrusts to a woman in the late stages of pregnancy whose airway is completely blocked. Then she begins to cough forcefully. You should—
    - ☐ a. Continue giving chest thrusts.
    - ☒ b. Stop giving chest thrusts.

Answers

9. **b.** You should give **chest thrusts** if the victim is greatly overweight or in the late stages of pregnancy.

10. **a.** When giving chest thrusts, place your fist **on the middle of the breastbone.**

11. **b.** You should **stop giving chest thrusts** if the victim begins to cough forcefully.

First Aid for an Unconscious Adult With a Complete Airway Obstruction

First aid for any unconscious victim begins with a primary survey. While checking the ABCs, you may find that the victim has an obstructed airway. The procedure for identifying a complete airway obstruction in an unconscious victim is given below. Start by surveying the scene, and then do a primary survey.

1. Check the victim for unresponsiveness.
2. Shout for help.
3. Position the victim on his or her back.
4. Open the airway.
5. Look, listen, and feel for breathing.
6. If the victim is not breathing, give 2 full breaths.
7. If you are unable to breathe air into the victim, retilt the head and give 2 full breaths. You may not have tilted the victim's head far enough back the first time.

If you still cannot breathe air into the victim, tell someone to phone the EMS system for help, and do the following steps:

8. Give 6 to 10 abdominal thrusts (as explained on the next page).
9. Do a finger sweep to try to dislodge and remove the object from the victim's throat (as explained on page 62).
10. Open the airway and give 2 full breaths.

Repeat steps 8, 9, and 10 until the obstruction is cleared or EMS personnel arrive and take over.

Abdominal Thrusts

To give abdominal thrusts—

- Straddle the victim's thighs *(Fig. 28)*.

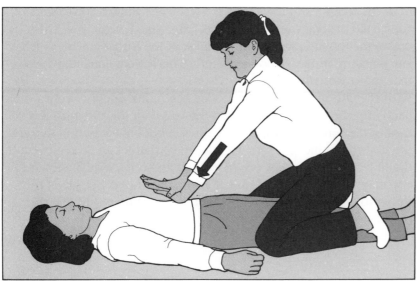

Figure 28
Abdominal Thrusts for Unconscious Victim

- Place the heel of one hand against the middle of the victim's abdomen, just above the navel and well below the lower tip of the breastbone *(Fig. 29)*. Place your other hand directly on top of the first hand with your fingers pointed toward the victim's head.
- Press into the abdomen with a quick upward thrust. Give 6 to 10 thrusts. Be sure that your hands are directly on the midline of the abdomen when you press. Do not direct the thrusts to the right or to the left. Each thrust should be a separate and distinct attempt to dislodge the object. After 6 to 10 thrusts, do a finger sweep.

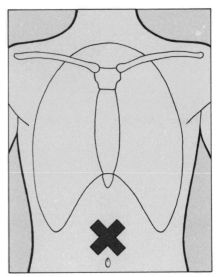

Figure 29
Location for Abdominal Thrusts

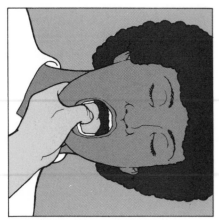

Figure 30
Grasp Tongue and Lower Jaw

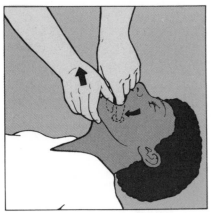

Figure 31
Finger Sweep

Finger Sweep

To do a finger sweep—

- Move from the straddle position and kneel beside the victim's head. Keeping the victim's face up, open the victim's mouth and grasp both the tongue and lower jaw between the thumb and fingers of your hand nearest the victim's legs *(Fig. 30)*. Lift the jaw. This draws the tongue away from the back of the throat and away from any object that may be lodged there. This action alone may help relieve the obstruction.
- With the jaw and tongue lifted, slide the index finger of your other hand into the mouth down along the inside of the throat to the base of the tongue *(Fig. 31)*. Then use a hooking action to dislodge the object and move it into the mouth so that it can be removed. If the object comes within reach, grasp it and remove it. Sometimes you may have to push the object against the opposite side of the throat to dislodge it and to lift it out. Be careful not to force the object deeper into the airway.

Review Questions

Check the best answer.

12. You encounter an unconscious victim who is not breathing. If you cannot breathe air into the victim's lungs on the first try, what should you do next?
   ☒ a. Retilt the head.
   ☐ b. Look in the mouth for an object blocking the airway.
   ☐ c. Give 6 to 10 abdominal thrusts.

13. When you are giving abdominal thrusts to an unconscious victim, you should—
   ☐ a. Kneel beside the victim's chest.
   ☐ b. Kneel by the victim's head.
   ☒ c. Straddle the victim's thighs.

14. To give abdominal thrusts to an unconscious victim, place the heel of one hand—
   ☐ a. Over the edge of the rib cage.
   ☒ b. In the middle of the victim's abdomen slightly above the navel and well below the lower tip of the breastbone.
   ☐ c. Directly over the navel.

15. In what direction should you give abdominal thrusts for an unconscious person?
   ☒ a. Upward
   ☐ b. Straight toward the ground

16. For an unconscious victim, how many abdominal thrusts should you give before doing a finger sweep?
   ☐ a. 15 to 20
   ☒ b. 6 to 10
   ☐ c. 1 to 3

17. When doing a finger sweep, try to remove the object by—
   ☒ a. Using a hooking action.
   ☐ b. Poking straight into the throat.

Answers

12. a. You should **retilt the head** if you cannot breathe air into the lungs of an unconscious victim who is not breathing.

13. c. You should **straddle the victim's thighs** when giving abdominal thrusts to an unconscious victim.

14. b. You should place the heel of one hand **in the middle of the victim's abdomen slightly above the navel and well below the lower tip of the breastbone** to give abdominal thrusts to an unconscious victim.

15. a. You should give abdominal thrusts **upward.**

16. b. You should give **6 to 10** abdominal thrusts before doing a finger sweep.

17. a. When doing a finger sweep, try to remove the object by **using a hooking action.**

Chest Thrusts for an Unconscious Adult

If an unconscious person with an obstructed airway is in the late stages of pregnancy or is greatly overweight, you should give chest thrusts.

You should follow the same steps as you would in giving first aid for choking to an unconscious adult, except that you give chest thrusts instead of abdominal thrusts. To give chest thrusts to an unconscious victim—

1. Kneel facing the victim.
2. Position your hands as you would if you were giving CPR chest compressions. You will learn how to do this in Chapter 5.
3. Give 6 to 10 thrusts. Each thrust should compress the chest 1½ to 2 inches (3.8 to 5 centimeters). Give slow and distinct thrusts as if you were trying to unblock the airway with each thrust.
4. Do a finger sweep.
5. Open the victim's airway and give 2 full breaths.

Repeat steps 3, 4, and 5 until the obstruction is cleared or EMS personnel arrive and take over.

Put the Steps Together

Here is the whole procedure for an unconscious adult who may have a complete airway obstruction:

1. Check for unresponsiveness.
2. Shout for help.
3. Position the victim on his or her back.
4. Open the airway.
5. Look, listen, and feel for breathing.
6. Give 2 full breaths.
7. Retilt the head if you are unable to breathe air into the victim.
8. Give 2 full breaths.
9. Have someone phone the EMS system for help if you are still unable to breathe air into the victim's lungs.
   Then do the next three steps.
10. Give 6 to 10 abdominal thrusts (or chest thrusts, if necessary).
11. Do a finger sweep.
12. Open the victim's airway and give 2 full breaths.

Repeat steps 10, 11, and 12 until the obstruction is cleared or EMS personnel arrive and take over.

If your first attempts to clear the airway are unsuccessful, **do not stop.** The longer the victim goes without oxygen, the more the muscles will relax, making it more likely that you will be able to clear the airway.

If you **are** able to breathe air into the victim's lungs, give 2 full breaths as you did for rescue breathing. Then check the pulse. If there is no pulse, begin CPR. (Chapter 5 describes CPR for an adult.) If there is a pulse and the victim is not breathing on his or her own, continue rescue breathing.

If the victim should start breathing on his or her own, monitor breathing and pulse until EMS personnel arrive and take over. This means you should maintain an open airway; look, listen, and feel for breathing; and keep checking the pulse. Keep the victim still.

Review Questions

Check the best answer.

18. You find a victim lying on the ground. You survey the scene and decide it is safe to help the victim. What should you do first?
    ☐ a. Open the airway.
    ☐ b. Begin rescue breathing.
    ☐ c. Check for unresponsiveness.

19. You find an unresponsive victim. You open the victim's airway and give 2 full breaths, but the air will not go in. What should you do next?
    ☐ a. Retilt the head.
    ☐ b. Do a finger sweep.
    ☐ c. Give 6 to 10 abdominal thrusts.

20. You retilt the head of an unconscious victim and give 2 more breaths. The air still does not go in. What should you do next?
    ☐ a. Open the airway.
    ☐ b. Do a finger sweep.
    ☐ c. Give 6 to 10 abdominal thrusts.

21. After doing a finger sweep, you find that the air you breathe into the victim goes into the lungs. You can see the victim's chest rise. What should you do next?
    ☐ a. Open the airway.
    ☐ b. Check the pulse.
    ☐ c. Phone the EMS system for help.

Answers

18. c. The first thing you should do if you find a victim lying on the ground is **check for unresponsiveness.**

19. a. If you are unable to breathe air into the victim's lungs on the first try, the next thing you should do is **retilt the head.**

20. c. If you are unable to breathe air into the victim's lungs on the second try, **give 6 to 10 abdominal thrusts.**

21. b. If you are able to breathe air into the victim's lungs, the next thing you should do is **check the pulse.**

First Aid for Choking When a Conscious Adult Becomes Unconscious

If an adult who is choking loses consciousness while you are giving abdominal or chest thrusts, you should shout for help and slowly lower the victim to the floor while supporting the victim from behind. Make sure the victim's head doesn't hit the floor.

Once you have lowered the victim to the floor, have someone phone the EMS system for help if it hasn't already been done. Then kneel beside the victim and do the following:

1. Do a finger sweep.
2. Open the airway and give 2 full breaths.
3. Give 6 to 10 abdominal thrusts if you are unable to breathe air into the victim's lungs.

Repeat these three steps in the same order until the obstruction is cleared or until EMS personnel arrive and take over.

Practice Session: First Aid for an Adult Who Is Choking (Complete Airway Obstruction)

During this practice session, you will practice on a partner, and then you will practice on a manikin.

Before you start practicing, carefully read the following directions and the skill sheets on pages 70 through 76. If you don't remember how to use the checklist, read pages 44 through 46.

In this practice session, you will learn two separate skills: first aid for a **conscious** adult with a complete airway obstruction, and first aid for an **unconscious** adult with a complete airway obstruction.

1. You will practice first aid for a conscious adult with a complete airway obstruction. You will practice this skill on a partner. If possible, a third person should read the skill sheet as you practice.

Remember: **When practicing abdominal thrusts on a partner, do not give actual abdominal thrusts.**

2. You will practice first aid for an unconscious adult with a complete airway obstruction. You will practice this skill on a manikin.

Remember: **Do not perform finger sweeps on a manikin. Do not touch the manikin's lips or inside the mouth with your fingers.**

Before you practice on the manikin, clean its face and the inside of its mouth. Directions for doing this are given in the section called "Some Health Precautions and Guidelines to Follow During This Course" on page 3 of this workbook. Clean the manikin's face and mouth before each person in your group practices.

Skill Sheet: First Aid for a Conscious Adult With a Complete Airway Obstruction

Remember: **When practicing abdominal thrusts on a partner, do not give actual abdominal thrusts.**

Partner Check

Instructor Check

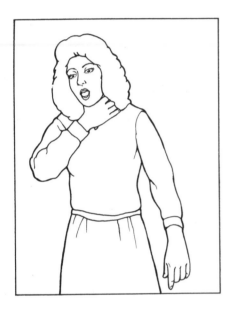

☐ ☑ **Determine If Victim Is Choking**

Rescuer asks, "Are you choking?"

Partner/Instructor says, "Victim cannot cough, speak, or breathe."

Rescuer shouts, "Help!"

☐ ☑ **Phone the EMS System for Help**

Tell someone to call for an ambulance.

Rescuer says, "Victim choking,
call_____."

(Local emergency number or Operator)

Partner Check
Instructor Check

☐ ☑ **Perform Abdominal Thrusts**

Stand behind victim.

Wrap arms around victim's waist.

Make a fist with one hand and place thumb side of fist against middle of victim's abdomen just above navel and well below lower tip of breastbone.

Grasp your fist with your other hand.

Keeping elbows out, press fist into victim's abdomen with a quick upward thrust.

Each thrust should be a separate and distinct attempt to dislodge the object.

Repeat thrusts until obstruction is cleared or victim becomes unconscious.

Final Instructor Check _____

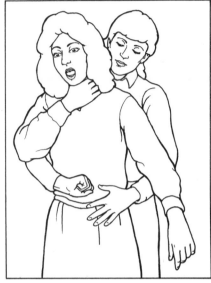

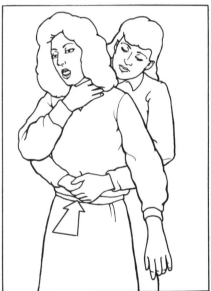

Skill Sheet: First Aid for an Unconscious Adult With a Complete Airway Obstruction

You find a person lying on the ground, not moving. You should survey the scene to see if it is safe and to get some idea of what happened. Then do a primary survey by checking the ABCs.

Remember: **Do not perform finger sweeps on a manikin. Do not touch the manikin's lips or inside the mouth with your fingers.**

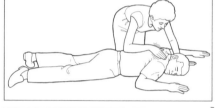

☐ ☑ **Check for Unresponsiveness**

Tap or gently shake victim.

Rescuer shouts, "Are you OK?"

Partner/Instructor says, "Unconscious."

Rescuer repeats, "Unconscious."

Rescuer shouts, "Help!"

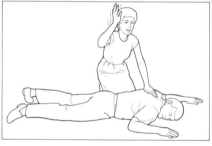

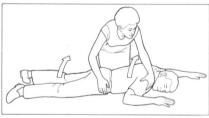

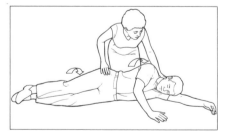

Position the Victim

Roll victim onto back, if necessary.

Kneel facing victim, midway between victim's hips and shoulders.

Straighten victim's legs, if necessary, and move victim's arm closest to you above victim's head.

Lean over victim, and place one hand on victim's shoulder and other hand on victim's hip.

Roll victim toward you as a single unit. As you roll victim, move your hand from victim's shoulder to support back of head and neck.

Place victim's arm closest to you alongside victim's body.

Partner Check
Instructor Check

☐ ☑ **Open the Airway** (Use head-tilt/chin-lift)

Place your hand—the one nearest the victim's head—on victim's forehead.

Place fingers of other hand under bony part of lower jaw near chin.

Tilt head and lift jaw. Avoid closing victim's mouth. Avoid pushing on the soft parts under the chin.

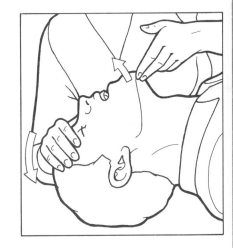

☐ ☑ **Check for Breathlessness**

Maintain open airway with head-tilt/chin-lift.

Place your ear over victim's mouth and nose.

Look at chest; listen and feel for breathing for 3 to 5 seconds.

Partner/Instructor says, "No breathing."

Rescuer repeats, "No breathing."

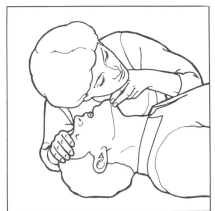

☐ ☑ **Give 2 Full Breaths**

Maintain open airway with head-tilt/chin-lift.

Pinch nose shut.

Open your mouth wide, take a deep breath, and seal your lips tightly around outside of victim's mouth.

Give 2 full breaths at the rate of 1 to 1½ seconds per breath. Pause between each breath for you to take a breath.

Partner/Instructor says, "Unable to breathe air into victim."

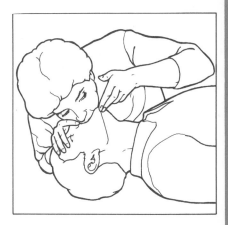

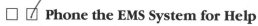

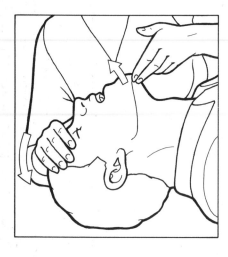

☐ ☑ **Retilt Victim's Head and Give 2 Full Breaths**

Retilt victim's head.

Pinch nose shut.

Open your mouth wide, take a deep breath, and seal your lips tightly around outside of victim's mouth.

Give 2 full breaths at the rate of 1 to 1½ seconds per breath. Pause between each breath for you to take a breath.

Partner/Instructor says, "Still unable to breathe air into victim."

Rescuer says, "Airway obstructed."

☐ ☑ **Phone the EMS System for Help**

Tell someone to call for an ambulance.

Rescuer says, "Airway obstructed, call_____."
(Local emergency number or Operator)

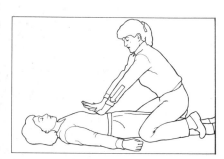

☐ ☑ **Perform 6 to 10 Abdominal Thrusts**

Straddle victim's thighs.

Place heel of one hand against middle of victim's abdomen just above navel and well below lower tip of breastbone.

Place other hand directly on top of first hand. (Fingers of both hands should be pointing toward victim's head.)

Press into victim's abdomen 6 to 10 times with quick upward thrusts.

Each thrust should be a separate and distinct attempt to dislodge the object.

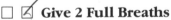

Partner Check

Instructor Check

☐ ☑ **Do Finger Sweep (Pretend)**

Move from straddle position and kneel beside victim's head.

With victim's face up, open the mouth and grasp both tongue and lower jaw between thumb and fingers of hand nearest victim's legs. Lift jaw.

Insert index finger into mouth along inside of cheek and deep into throat to base of tongue.

Use "hooking" action to dislodge object and move it into mouth for removal.

Partner/Instructor says, "No object found."

Rescuer repeats, "No object found."

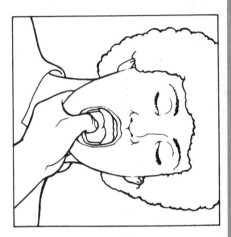

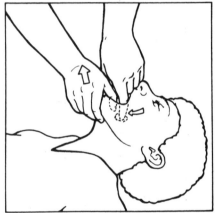

☐ ☑ **Give 2 Full Breaths**

Open airway with head-tilt/chin-lift.

Pinch nose shut.

Open your mouth wide, take a deep breath, and seal your lips tightly around outside of victim's mouth.

Give 2 full breaths at the rate of 1 to 1½ seconds per breath. Pause between each breath for you to take a breath.

Partner/Instructor says, "Airway still obstructed."

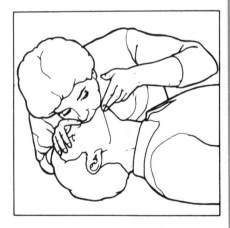

Partner Check

Instructor Check

☐ ☑ **Repeat Sequence**

Do 6 to 10 abdominal thrusts.

Do finger sweep (pretend).

Give 2 full breaths.

☐ ☑ **What to Do Next**

While the rescuer is repeating the sequence of abdominal thrusts, finger sweep, and rescue breaths, the partner should read one of the following statements:

1. Rescuer can breathe into victim's lungs after doing finger sweep.

2. Object is removed during finger sweep.

3. Object is expelled during abdominal thrusts.

Based on this information, the rescuer should decide what to do next and continue giving the right care.

Final Instructor Check *MER*

4 *What to Do for Heart Attack*

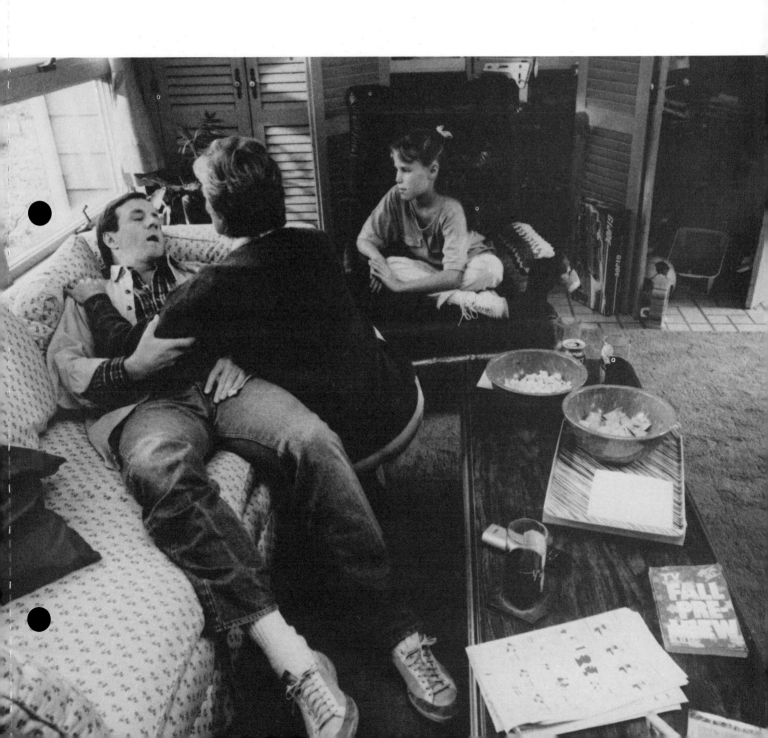

*In this chapter, you will learn what a heart attack is and what to do for someone who is having a heart attack. You will also learn what you can do to prevent heart attacks. To give a heart attack victim the best chance of surviving, you must first be able to **recognize** the signals of a heart attack. This isn't always easy. Once you recognize the signals, you must then give the correct first aid.*

Objectives

By the time you finish reading this chapter, you should be able to do the following:

1. List three signals of a heart attack.

2. Describe why it is important to know that heart attack victims often deny that they are having a heart attack.

3. Describe the first aid for a heart attack.

4. List the risk factors for cardiovascular disease.

What Is a Heart Attack?

A heart attack happens when one or more of the blood vessels that supply blood to a portion of the heart become blocked. When this happens, the blood can't get through to feed that part of the heart. When the flow of oxygen-carrying blood is cut off, the cells of this part of the heart begin to die. This is what happens during a heart attack. The heart may not be able to pump properly because part of it is dying.

If a large part of the heart is not getting blood, then the heart may not be able to pump at all. If the heart stops, it is called **cardiac arrest**.

Since any heart attack may lead to cardiac arrest, it is important to be able to recognize when someone is having a heart attack. Prompt action may prevent the victim's heart from stopping. The simple truth is that a heart attack victim whose heart is still beating has a far better chance of living than someone whose heart has stopped. Most people who die from a heart attack die within one to two hours after the first signals of the heart attack occur. Many of these people could be saved if bystanders were able to recognize the signals of a heart attack and take prompt action.

Signals of a Heart Attack

The most significant signal of a heart attack is chest discomfort or pain. A victim may describe it as uncomfortable pressure, squeezing, a fullness or tightness, or as an aching, crushing, constricting, oppressive, or heavy feeling. The pain is described as being in the center of the chest behind the breastbone. The pain may spread to one or both shoulders or arms, or to the neck, jaw, or back *(Fig. 32)*.

In addition to chest pain, there may be other signals, including—

- Sweating.
- Nausea.
- Shortness of breath.

Many victims deny that they are having a heart attack. They may not want to admit to themselves or to others that they are having a heart attack. This may delay medical care when it is needed most. Heart attack victims may deny that they are having a heart attack by saying, for example, "I'm too healthy," or "It's indigestion or something I ate," or "It can't happen to me," or "I don't want to bother my doctor," or "This is something I can take care of myself," or "I don't want to frighten anyone," or "I'll feel ridiculous bothering everybody if it isn't a heart attack." These excuses are a signal to take immediate action.

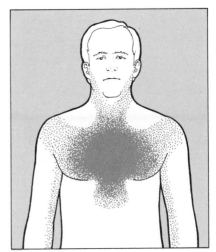

Figure 32
Areas for Heart Attack Pain

First Aid for Heart Attacks

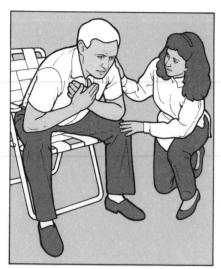

Figure 33
Caring for the Heart Attack Victim

To give first aid for a heart attack, you should—
1. Recognize the signals of a heart attack and take action.
2. Have the person stop what he or she is doing and sit or lie down in a comfortable position. Do not let the victim move around.
3. Have someone phone the emergency medical services (EMS) system for help. If you are alone with the victim, you should make the call.

A key factor in whether or not a victim will survive a heart attack is how quickly the victim receives advanced care. Therefore, it is important that you call the EMS system right away.

Not all ambulances are staffed and equipped to provide advanced care to the victim at the scene of an emergency, but in most cases it is better to call for an ambulance to transport the victim rather than to transport the victim in a private vehicle yourself. The victim's condition could worsen on the way to the hospital, and an ambulance is equipped and staffed to deal with conditions that could develop during the transport. In addition, transporting a victim in a private vehicle places tremendous emotional pressures on the driver. This puts **all** occupants of the vehicle at added risk.

There may be some situations, however, when an ambulance is not readily available, and you may have to weigh the risks and consider driving the victim to the hospital. You should know that not all hospitals and health facilities offer advanced care for cardiac emergencies, and of those that do, not all of them offer it on a 24-hour basis. Therefore, it is important to be familiar with the emergency resources of your community and make a plan of action **before** an emergency happens.

After the EMS system has been called, you should ask the victim for information about his or her condition *(Fig. 33).* Bystanders may also be able to give you some of this information. The questions you should ask as part of this interview are explained in Chapter 1. You should try to get the following information:
- Victim's name
- Victim's age
- Previous medical problems ("Has anything like this ever happened to you before?")
- Where it hurts and how long the person has had pain
- Type of pain (for example, "dull," "heavy," "sharp")

Because the heart attack victim's heart may stop beating, you should be prepared to give CPR.

Review Questions

Fill in the blanks with the right word or check the best answer.

1. What is the most significant signal of a heart attack?
   _____ or _____

2. What is the first aid for a heart attack?
   a. Recognize the _____ of a heart attack.
   b. Make the victim _____ or _____ down in a comfortable position.
   c. Call the _____ system for help.

3. As you are walking home from work, you notice your neighbor sitting in her car in her driveway. She explains that she is having pain in her chest and asks you to help her into her house. Which of the following should you **not** do, if possible?
   ☐ a. Help her walk to the house.
   ☐ b. Tell her to rest where she is.

Answers

1. The most significant signal of a heart attack is **chest discomfort** or **chest pain.**

2. The first aid for a heart attack is to—
   a. Recognize the **signals** of a heart attack.
   b. Make the victim **sit** or **lie** down in a comfortable position.
   c. Call the **EMS** system for help.

3. a. You should **not help her walk to the house**. (A person who is having chest pain should not move around.)

How Heart Attacks Happen

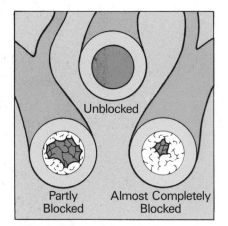

Figure 34
Blocked Arteries

While heart attacks seem to strike suddenly, the conditions that often cause them may build up silently for years. Most heart attacks are the result of **cardiovascular disease**. Cardiovascular disease happens when fatty substances and other materials build up in the blood and begin to stick to the walls of the blood vessels. Over time, the blood vessels get narrower. As the blood vessels get narrower, it becomes more and more likely that a blood vessel in the heart will become partly or completely clogged *(Fig. 34)*. This process can begin in early life; some scientists believe it may even begin in early childhood.

Most of the people in this room may have some form of cardiovascular disease. Cardiovascular disease may only be stopped or slowed by certain changes in the way you live. This disease cannot be stopped by medicines, though some related problems (like high blood pressure) can be controlled or slowed by medicines.

Risk Factors

Scientists have been able to identify certain things that are related to getting cardiovascular disease. They call these **risk factors**. In this course, there is not enough time to give you a lot of information about risk factors, but we have included the list below so that you can see which apply to you:

• **Risk factors that you cannot change are—**
  • Heredity (a history of cardiovascular disease in your family).
  • Sex (males are at greater risk).
  • Age (you are at greater risk as you get older).

- **Risk factors that you can change are—**
  - Cigarette smoking.
  - High blood pressure.
  - High blood cholesterol (influenced by a diet high in saturated fat and cholesterol).
  - Uncontrolled diabetes.
  - Obesity (being overweight).
  - Lack of exercise.
  - Stress.

You **can** reduce your risk of cardiovascular disease. But, it will take effort on your part and guidance from your doctor or health care provider. If you want to learn more about how to reduce your risk of having a heart attack, the American Red Cross can tell you about resources available in your community to help you.

Review Questions

Fill in the blanks with the right word.

4. When a person has cardiovascular disease, over time that person's blood vessels get _____.

5. Blood vessels become clogged when _____ substances and other materials begin to stick to the walls of the blood vessels.

6. Most heart attacks happen when blood vessels become clogged and cut off the flow of _____ to the heart.

7. What are the risk factors for cardiovascular disease that you cannot change?
   a. Heredity (a history of cardiovascular disease in your _____).
   b. Sex (_____ are at greater risk).
   c. Age (you are at greater risk as you get _____).

8. What are seven risk factors that you can work on to reduce your risk of cardiovascular disease?
   a. Cigarette smoking
   b. _____ blood pressure
   c. High blood cholesterol
   d. Lack of _____
   e. Obesity or being _____
   f. Uncontrolled diabetes
   g. Stress

Answers

4. When a person has cardiovascular disease, over time that person's blood vessels get **narrower**.

5. Blood vessels become clogged when **fatty** substances and other materials begin to stick to the walls of the blood vessels.

6. Most heart attacks happen when blood vessels become clogged and cut off the flow of **blood** to the heart.

7. The risk factors for cardiovascular disease that you cannot change are—
   a. Heredity (a history of cardiovascular disease in your **family**).
   b. Sex (**males** are at greater risk).
   c. Age (you are at greater risk as you get **older**).

8. Seven risk factors that you can work on to reduce your risk of cardiovascular disease are—
   a. Cigarette smoking.
   b. **High** blood pressure.
   c. High blood cholesterol.
   d. Lack of **exercise.**
   e. Obesity or being **overweight.**
   f. Uncontrolled diabetes.
   g. Stress.

5 What to Do When an Adult's Heart Stops (CPR)

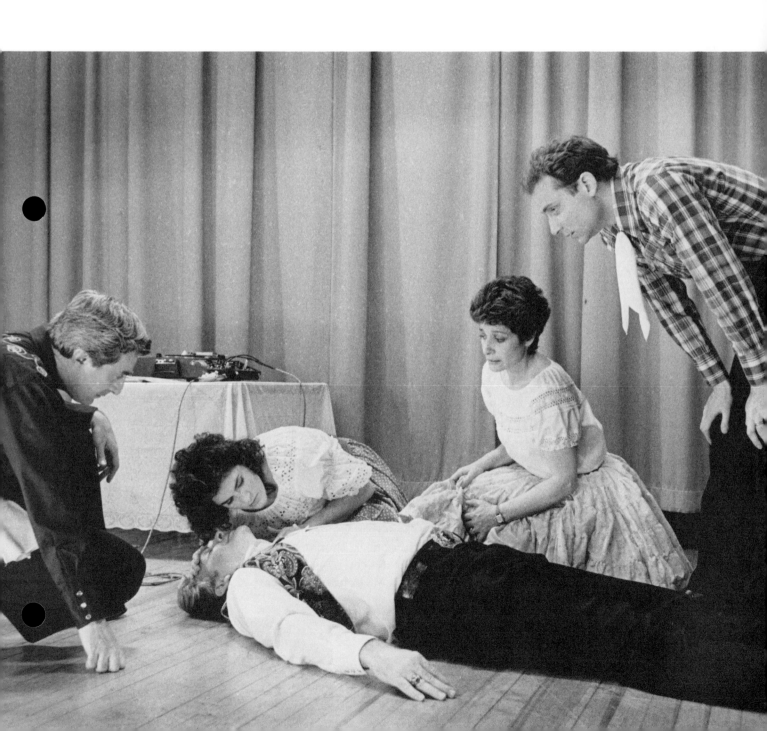

In this chapter, you will find out what to do for an adult whose heart has stopped beating. You will learn how to keep oxygen-carrying blood moving through the victim's body.

Cardiopulmonary resuscitation (CPR) is a combination of chest compressions and rescue breathing. "Cardio" refers to the heart and "pulmonary" refers to the lungs. When you give CPR, you do chest compressions and rescue breathing together. This supplies oxygen to the victim's blood and moves the blood through the body to supply the cells with oxygen. If a person's heart stops for any reason, CPR must be started immediately. To have the best chance to survive, the person must receive advanced emergency medical care within 10 minutes.

Objectives

By the time you finish reading this chapter, you should be able to do the following:
1. *Describe the location and function of the heart.*
2. *Describe the purpose of CPR (cardiopulmonary resuscitation).*
3. *Explain why it is important to check the victim's carotid pulse before you start CPR.*
4. *Describe how to do CPR on an adult.*
5. *Describe when you should check for the return of the victim's pulse after you start CPR.*
6. *List four conditions when a rescuer may stop CPR.*

A Look at the Heart

The heart is a tough muscular organ about the size of your fist. It is located roughly in the center of your chest between the lungs and under the lower half of the breastbone. The heart is protected in the front by the ribs and breastbone and in the back by the backbone.

The heart pumps blood to all parts of your body through blood vessels. Blood vessels are the tubes that carry blood to the cells of the body. How well this system works depends on the condition of your blood vessels and your heart *(Fig. 35).*

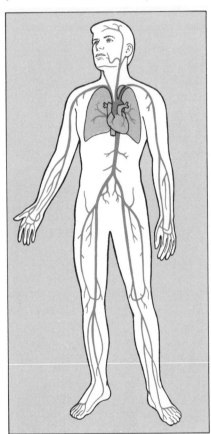

Figure 35
The Heart and Major Blood Vessels

For the average adult, the heart pumps about 70 times each minute, or about 100,000 times each day. In the minute or so it takes you to read this section, your heart will pump more than a gallon of blood. If a person's heart should stop beating, that person would need help immediately to keep oxygen-carrying blood flowing to the body's cells until EMS personnel arrive.

Review Questions

Fill in the blanks with the right word.

1. The purpose of the heart is to __pump__ blood to all parts of the body.

2. How well your circulatory system works depends on the condition of your __heart__ and your blood __vessels__.

Answers

1. The purpose of the heart is to **pump** blood to all parts of the body.

2. How well your circulatory system works depends on the condition of your **heart** and your blood **vessels.**

The Purpose of CPR and Why It Works

To help a person in cardiac arrest, you must provide CPR. CPR has two purposes. By breathing into the victim and compressing the chest, you—

1. Keep the lungs supplied with oxygen when breathing has stopped.
2. Keep blood circulating and carrying oxygen to the brain, heart, and other parts of the body.

All of the body's living cells need a steady supply of oxygen to maintain life. CPR must be started as soon as possible after the heart stops. Any delay in starting CPR reduces the chances that EMS personnel will be able to restart the heart. In addition, brain cells begin to die after 4 to 6 minutes without oxygen.

Review Questions

Fill in the blanks with the right word.

3. The two purposes of CPR are—
   a. To keep the lungs supplied with _oxygen_ when breathing has stopped.
   b. To keep _blood_ circulating and carrying _oxygen_ to the brain, heart, and other parts of the body.

4. CPR must be started as soon as possible to increase the chances that EMS personnel will be able to _restart_ the heart.

Answers

3. The two purposes of CPR are—
   a. To keep the lungs supplied with **oxygen** when breathing has stopped.
   b. To keep **blood** circulating and carrying **oxygen** to the brain, heart, and other parts of the body.

4. CPR must be started as soon as possible to increase the chances that EMS personnel will be able to **restart** the heart.

How to Give CPR to an Adult

To find out if a person needs CPR, begin with a primary survey to check the ABCs as you did for rescue breathing. You should—
1. Check for unresponsiveness.
2. Shout for help.
3. Position the victim on his or her back.
4. Open the airway.
5. Look, listen, and feel for breathing.
6. If the person is not breathing, give 2 full breaths.
7. Check the carotid pulse.
8. Have someone phone the EMS system for help.

 If the victim has no pulse, begin CPR. **It is important to check the victim's carotid pulse for 5 to 10 seconds before you start CPR because it is dangerous to do chest compressions if the victim's heart is beating**.

To give CPR, kneel beside the victim, lean over the chest, and find the correct position to give chest compressions. Give chest compressions by pressing down and letting up at a steady pace. Then give rescue breaths. These two steps keep oxygen-carrying blood flowing through the blood vessels.

Locating the Compression Position

For chest compressions to work, the victim must be lying flat on his or her back on a firm, flat surface. The victim's head must be on the same level as the heart.

To give effective compressions, your hands and body must be in the correct position. Do the following:

- Kneel facing the victim's chest with your knees against the victim's side.
- Use your hand—the one nearest the victim's legs—to find the lower edge of the rib cage on the side closest to you. Slide your middle and index fingers up the edge of the rib cage to the notch where the ribs meet the breastbone in the center of the lower part of the chest *(Fig. 36)*. With your middle finger on this notch, place the index finger of the same hand next to it on the lower end of the breastbone.
- Place the heel of your other hand on the breastbone right next to the index finger of the hand you used to find the notch. The heel of your hand should rest along the length of the breastbone *(Fig. 37)*.

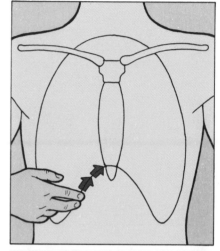

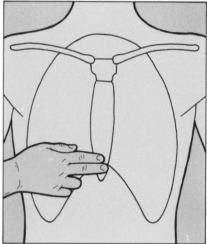

Figure 36
Find Correct Position

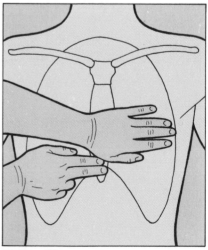

Figure 37
Place Heel of Hand on Breastbone

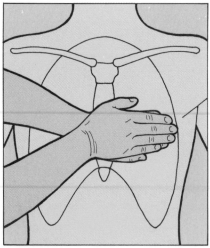

Figure 38
Place Second Hand Over Heel of First

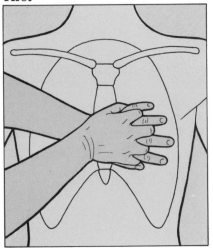

Figure 39
Interlace Fingers

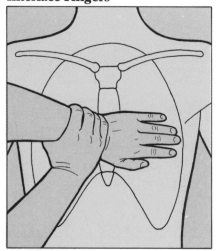

Figure 40
Alternate Hand Placement

- Once the heel of your hand is in position on the chest, remove the other hand from the notch and place the heel of this hand directly on top of the heel of the hand already on the victim's breastbone *(Fig. 38)*.
- Keep your fingers off the victim's chest. To do this, you may interlace them or hold them upward *(Fig. 39)*.
- Finding the correct hand position in this way allows you to compress right on the breastbone, and keeps hand pressure off the ribs and away from the tip of the breastbone. This will decrease the chance of fracturing the ribs, which are on either side of the breastbone. It will also keep you from pushing the tip of the breastbone into the delicate organs beneath it.
- Another acceptable hand position, useful for people with arthritic conditions, is made by grasping the wrist of the hand on the chest with the other hand *(Fig. 40)*.

Review Questions

Check the best answer(s).

5. Which of the following surfaces would be good for a victim to be on when you give CPR? (Check all that apply.)
   - ☐ a. Bed
   - ☑ b. Floor
   - ☑ c. Ground

6. The first step in finding the proper hand position for giving chest compressions is to—
   - ☑ a. Slide your middle and index fingers up the edge of the rib cage to the notch where the ribs meet the breastbone.
   - ☐ b. Find the top of the breastbone.
   - ☐ c. Find the navel.

7. When your hands are in the correct position to give CPR, where should your fingers be?
   - ☐ a. Resting on the victim's chest.
   - ☑ b. Held off the victim's chest.
   - ☐ c. Curling into your palm.

Answers

5. When you give CPR, the victim should be on a firm, flat surface such as the—
   b. Floor, or
   c. Ground.

6. a. The first step in finding the proper hand position for giving chest compressions is to **slide your middle and index fingers up the edge of the rib cage to the notch where the ribs meet the breastbone.**

7. b. When your hands are in the correct position to give CPR, your fingers should be **held off the victim's chest.**

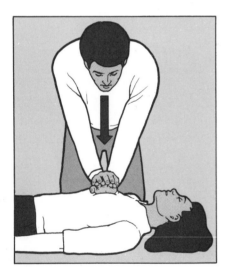

Figure 41
Correct Position of Rescuer

Body Position of the Rescuer

The position of your body is very important when you are giving compressions. You should be kneeling facing the victim's chest and have your hands in the correct position. Straighten your arms and lock your elbows so that your shoulders are directly over your hands. In this position when you push down, you will be pushing straight down onto the breastbone. The weight of your upper body creates the pressure necessary to compress the chest *(Fig. 41).*

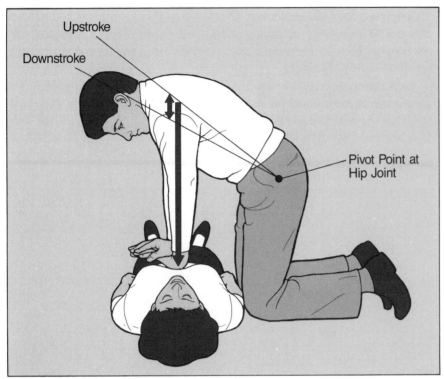

Figure 42
Giving Chest Compressions

Compression Technique

This is how you give chest compressions to an adult:

1. When you compress, push with the weight of your body, not with the muscles of your arms. Push straight down. If you rock back and forth and don't push straight down, your compressions will not be effective *(Fig. 42)*.
2. Each compression should push the breastbone down from 1½ to 2 inches (3.8 to 5 centimeters) *(Fig. 43)*.

The downward and upward movement should be smooth, not jerky. Maintain a steady down-and-up rhythm and do not pause between compressions. Half the time should be spent pushing down, and half the time should be spent coming up. When you are coming up, release pressure on the chest completely, but don't let your hands lose contact with the chest or lose their correct position on the breastbone.

3. Give compressions at the rate of 80 to 100 compressions per minute.
4. If your hands lose contact with the chest, find the compression position again before you start compressing. Find the notch as you did before, in order to position your hands correctly.

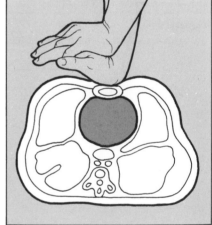

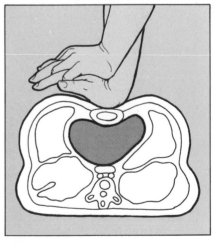

Figure 43
Compress Chest 1½ to 2 Inches

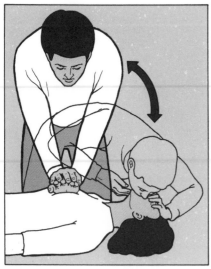

Figure 44
15 Compressions, Then 2 Breaths

Compression/Breathing Cycles

When you give CPR, do cycles of 15 compressions and 2 breaths. In each cycle, give 15 compressions and then open the airway and give 2 full breaths *(Fig. 44)*.

Each time you begin a new cycle of compressions and breaths, locate the correct hand position for compressions by finding the notch at the lower end of the breastbone.

Review Questions

Check the best answer.

8. When you give CPR, your arms should be—
- ☐ a. Bent.
- ☒ b. Straight.

9. How far should you compress the chest of an adult?
- ☐ a. 1 to 1½ inches (2.5 to 3.8 centimeters)
- ☒ b. 1½ to 2 inches (3.8 to 5 centimeters)
- ☐ c. 2 to 3 inches (5 to 7.6 centimeters)

10. At what rate should you compress the chest during CPR?
- ☐ a. 50 to 60 times per minute
- ☐ b. 60 to 80 times per minute
- ☒ c. 80 to 100 times per minute

11. What should you do if your hands move out of position while compressing the chest?
- ☐ a. Continue compressions.
- ☒ b. Reposition your hands by locating the notch and continue compressions.
- ☐ c. Place your hands back where they were but do not waste time by relocating the notch.

15 compressions & 2 breaths

Do 4 complete cycles

Answers

8. b. When you give CPR, your arms should be **straight**.

9. b. You should compress the chest of an adult **1½ to 2 inches** (3.8 to 5 centimeters).

10. c. During CPR, you should compress the chest at the rate of **80 to 100 times per minute**.

11. b. If your hands move out of position, **reposition your hands by locating the notch and continue compressions**.

Put the Steps Together

Here are the steps you should follow when you give CPR to an adult:

1. Check for unresponsiveness. Tap or gently shake the person and shout, "Are you OK?"
2. Shout for help.
3. Position the victim.
4. Open the airway.
5. Look, listen, and feel for breathing (3 to 5 seconds).
6. If the victim is not breathing, give 2 full breaths.
7. Check the victim's carotid pulse for heartbeat (5 to 10 seconds).
8. Tell someone to phone the EMS system for help.
9. If there is no pulse, find the correct hand position and position your body to give compressions.
10. Give 15 compressions without stopping, at the rate of 80 to 100 per minute, counting out loud, "One and two and three and four and five and six and seven and eight and nine and ten and eleven and twelve and thirteen and fourteen and fifteen and." Push down as you say the number and come up as you say the "and."
11. Quickly tilt the victim's head back and lift the jaw. Give 2 full breaths to the victim the same way you gave the first 2 breaths.
12. Keep repeating—15 compressions, 2 breaths, 15 compressions, 2 breaths, and so on. The complete cycle of 15 compressions and 2 breaths should take from 11 to 14 seconds.
13. Recheck pulse. After doing 4 cycles (or about 1 minute) of continuous CPR, check to see if the victim has a pulse. Do this after giving the 2 breaths at the end of the 4th cycle of 15 compressions and 2 breaths. Tilt the victim's head back and check the carotid pulse for 5 seconds. If there is no pulse, give 2 breaths and continue CPR (compressions and rescue breaths). Repeat these pulse checks every few minutes.

If you do find a pulse, then check for breathing for 3 to 5 seconds. If breathing is present, keep the airway open and monitor breathing and pulse closely. This means that you should look, listen, and feel for breathing while you keep checking the pulse. If there is no breathing, do rescue breathing and keep checking the pulse.

14. Continue CPR until one of the following things happens:
    - The heart starts beating again.
    - A second rescuer trained in CPR takes over for you.
    - EMS personnel arrive and take over.
    - You are too exhausted to continue.

Review Questions

Check the best answer or fill in the blanks with the right word.

12. When you give CPR, what is the ratio of compressions to breaths?
    - ☐ a. 10 compressions, then 1 breath
    - ☑ b. 15 compressions, then 2 breaths
    - ☐ c. 12 compressions, then 15 breaths

13. After starting CPR, how often should you check for the return of pulse?
    - ☐ a. After 5 minutes and every 5 to 6 minutes thereafter
    - ☐ b. After 2 minutes and every 4 to 5 minutes thereafter
    - ☑ c. After 1 minute and every few minutes thereafter

14. What are the four conditions when you may stop CPR?
    a. When the heart starts _beating_ again.
    b. When a second rescuer trained in _CPR_ takes over for you.
    c. When _EMS_ personnel arrive and take over.
    d. When you are too _exhausted_ to continue.

Answers

12. **b.** When you give CPR, the ratio is **15 compressions, then 2 breaths**.

13. **c.** After starting CPR, you should check for the return of pulse **after 1 minute and every few minutes thereafter**.

14. You may stop CPR—
    a. When the heart starts **beating** again.
    b. When a second rescuer trained in **CPR** takes over for you.
    c. When **EMS** personnel arrive and take over.
    d. When you are too **exhausted** to continue.

More About CPR for an Adult

If No One Comes When You Shout for Help

One of the first things you do when you find an unresponsive victim is to shout for help. You do this to attract the attention of someone nearby who can phone the EMS system for help. But what if no one responds to your shouts for help? You should do CPR for at least 1 minute. During this minute you should continue to shout for help whenever you can. You should also use this minute to plan how to make the call yourself.

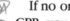 If no one answers your shouts for help by the end of 1 minute of
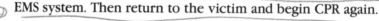 CPR, you should get to a phone as quickly as you can and phone the EMS system. Then return to the victim and begin CPR again.

If a Second Trained Rescuer Is at the Scene

If another rescuer trained in CPR is at the scene, this person should do two things: first, phone the EMS system for help if this has not been done; second, take over CPR when the first rescuer is tired. Here are the steps for entry of the second rescuer:

- The second person should first identify himself or herself as a CPR-trained rescuer who is willing to help.
- If the EMS system has been called and if the first rescuer is tired and asks for help, then—

    1. The first rescuer should stop CPR after the next set of 2 breaths.

    2. The second rescuer should kneel next to the victim opposite the first rescuer, tilt the head back, and feel for the carotid pulse for 5 seconds.

    3. If there is no pulse, the second rescuer should give 2 breaths and continue CPR.

4. The first rescuer should then check the adequacy of the second rescuer's breaths and chest compressions. This is done by watching the victim's chest rise and fall during rescue breathing and by feeling the carotid pulse for an artificial pulse during chest compressions. This artificial pulse will tell you that blood is moving through the body.

Practice Session: CPR for an Adult

During this practice session, you and a partner will practice only on a manikin.

Before you start practicing, carefully read the skill sheet on pages 102 through 109. If you don't remember how to use the checklist, read pages 44 through 46.

Before you practice on the manikin, clean its face and the inside of its mouth. Directions for doing this are given in the section called "Some Health Precautions and Guidelines to Follow During This Course" on page 3 of this workbook. Clean the manikin's face and mouth before each person in your group practices.

Skill Sheet: CPR for an Adult

You find a person lying on the ground, not moving. You should survey the scene to see if it is safe and to get some idea of what happened. Then do a primary survey by checking the ABCs.

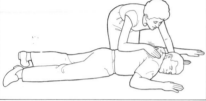

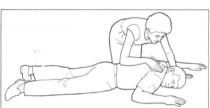

Check for Unresponsiveness

Tap or gently shake victim.

Rescuer shouts, "Are you OK?"

Partner/Instructor says, "Unconscious."
Rescuer repeats, "Unconscious."

Rescuer shouts, "Help!"

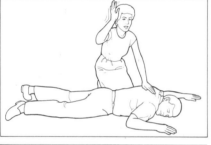

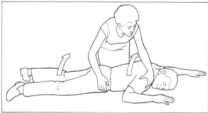

Position the Victim

Roll victim onto back, if necessary.

Kneel facing victim, midway between victim's hips and shoulders.

Straighten victim's legs, if necessary, and move victim's arm closest to you above victim's head.

Lean over victim, and place one hand on victim's shoulder and other hand on victim's hip.

Roll victim toward you as a single unit. As you roll victim, move your hand from victim's shoulder to support back of head and neck.

Place victim's arm closest to you alongside victim's body.

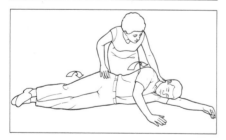

☐ ☐ **Open the Airway** (Use head-tilt/chin-lift)

Place your hand—the one nearest the victim's head—on victim's forehead.

Place fingers of other hand under bony part of lower jaw near chin.

Tilt head and lift jaw. Avoid closing victim's mouth. Avoid pushing on the soft parts under the chin.

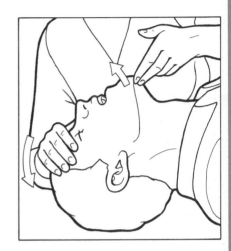

☐ ☑ **Check for Breathlessness**

Maintain open airway with head-tilt/chin-lift.

Place your ear over victim's mouth and nose.

Look at chest; listen and feel for breathing for 3 to 5 seconds.

Partner/Instructor says, "No breathing."

Rescuer repeats, "No breathing."

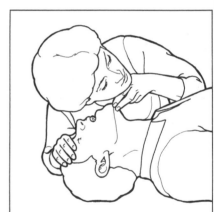

☐ ☑ **Give 2 Full Breaths**

Maintain open airway with head-tilt/chin-lift.

Pinch nose shut.

Open your mouth wide, take a deep breath, and seal your lips tightly around outside of victim's mouth.

Give 2 full breaths at the rate of 1 to 1½ seconds per breath. Pause between each breath for you to take a breath.

Look for the chest to rise and fall; listen and feel for escaping air.

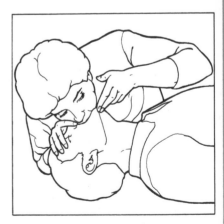

Partner Check
Instructor Check

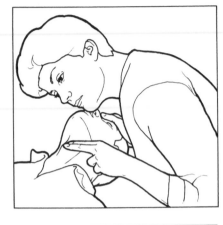

☐ ☑ **Check for Pulse**

Maintain head-tilt with one hand on forehead.

Locate Adam's apple with middle and index fingers of hand nearest victim's feet.

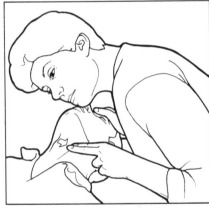

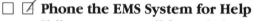

Slide fingers down into groove of neck on side closest to you.

Feel for carotid pulse for 5 to 10 seconds.

Partner/Instructor says, "No breathing and no pulse."

Rescuer repeats, "No breathing and no pulse."

☐ ☑ **Phone the EMS System for Help**

Tell someone to call for ambulance.

Rescuer says, "No breathing, no pulse, call ＿＿＿＿＿＿＿."

(*Local emergency number or Operator*)

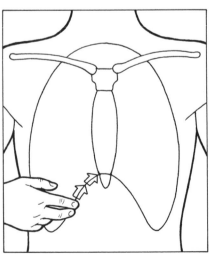

☐ ☑ **Locate Compression Position**

Kneel facing victim's chest.

With middle and index fingers of hand nearest victim's legs, locate lower edge of victim's rib cage on side closest to you.

Slide fingers up edge of rib cage to notch at lower end of breastbone.

Place middle finger in notch, and index finger next to it on the lower end of breastbone.

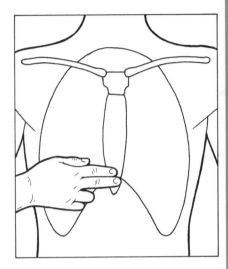

Place heel of hand nearest victim's head on breastbone next to index finger of hand used to find notch.

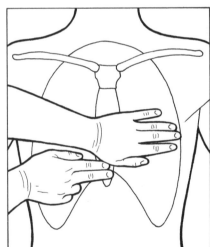

Place heel of hand used to locate notch directly on top of heel of other hand.

Keep fingers off victim's chest.

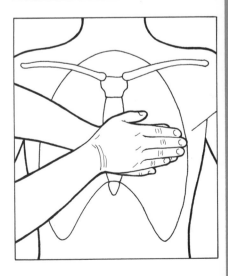

Partner Check
Instructor Check

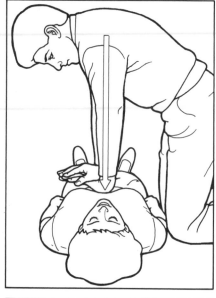

Position shoulders over hands with elbows locked and arms straight.

☐ ☑ **Give 15 Compressions**

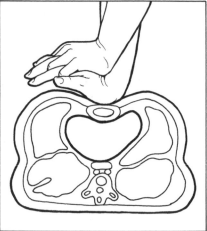

Compress breastbone 1½ to 2 inches (3.8 to 5 centimeters) at a rate of 80 to 100 compressions per minute. (15 compressions should take 9 to 11 seconds.)

Count aloud, "One and two and three and four and five and six and . . . fifteen and." (Push down as you say the number and come up as you say "and.")

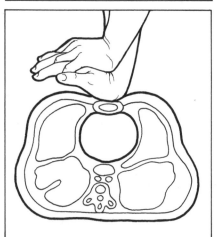

Compress down and up smoothly, keeping hand contact with chest at all times.

Partner Check
Instructor Check

☐ ☐ **Give 2 Full Breaths**
Open airway with head-tilt/chin-lift.

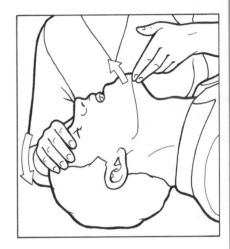

Pinch nose shut.

Open your mouth wide, take a deep breath, and seal your lips tightly around outside of victim's mouth.

Give 2 full breaths at the rate of 1 to 1½ seconds per breath. Pause between each breath for you to take a breath.

Look for chest to rise and fall; listen and feel for escaping air.

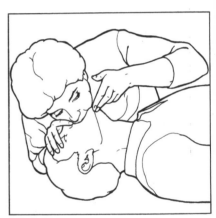

☐ ☑ **Do Compression/Breathing Cycles**
Do 4 cycles of 15 compressions and 2 breaths.

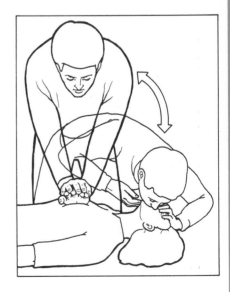

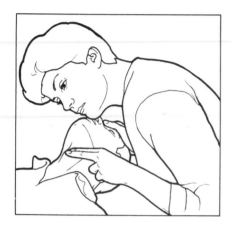

Partner Check   Instructor Check

☐ ☑ **Recheck Pulse**
Tilt head.

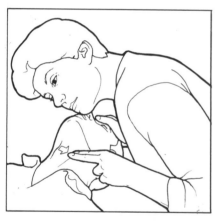

Locate carotid pulse and feel for 5 seconds.

Partner/Instructor says, "No pulse."

Rescuer repeats, "No pulse."

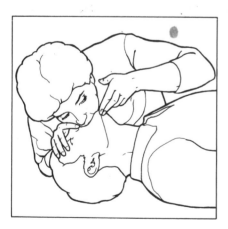

☐ ☐ **Give 2 Full Breaths**
Open airway with head-tilt/chin-lift.

Pinch nose shut.

Open your mouth wide, take a deep breath, and seal your lips tightly around outside of victim's mouth.

Give 2 full breaths at the rate of 1 to 1½ seconds per breath.

Look for the chest to rise and fall; listen and feel for escaping air.

□ ☑ **Continue Compression/Breathing Cycles**

Locate correct hand position.

Continue cycles of 15 compressions and 2 breaths.

Recheck pulse every few minutes.

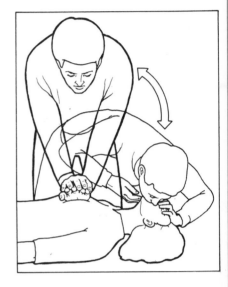

□ ☑ **What to Do Next**

When the rescuer stops to check pulse, the partner should read one of the following statements:

1. Victim has a pulse.

2. Victim does not have a pulse.

Based on this information, the rescuer should decide what to do next and continue giving the right care.

Final Instructor Check _MEλ._

Review Questions for Unit One

Directions

This section will help you review what you have learned in Unit One. You will be presented with a number of situations that you may find in real life. Fill in the blanks to tell what you would do if you came across these situations. The clues will help you make the correct decisions about what you should do.

Review Question: Rescue Breathing for an Adult

You are walking by your neighbor's house, and you hear shouts for help coming from the backyard. You run to the back of his house, and as you begin to survey the scene, you find your neighbor on the pool deck leaning over his wife. She is stretched out on her back and is not moving. Your neighbor says he found his wife at the bottom of the pool and pulled her out. What would you do next?

Do a primary survey to check the ABCs.

1. Check for _responsiveness_. (See clue below.)

2. Shout for _help_.

3. Open the _airway_.

4. Look, listen, and feel for _breath_. (See clue.)

5. Give 2 full _breath_.

6. Check for a _pulse_ at the side of the _neck_. (See clue.)

7. Have someone phone the _EMS system_ for help.

8. Begin _rescue breathing_.

9. Give 1 breath every _five_ seconds. (See clue.)

10. Keep the victim from moving until _rescue_ personnel arrive, and keep checking the victim's _breathing_ and _pulse_.

CLUES: • At step 1, the victim is unconscious.
   • At step 4, the victim is not breathing.
   • At step 6, the victim has a pulse.
   • At step 9, after you have given rescue breaths for 2 minutes, the victim begins to breathe on her own.

Answers

1. Check for **unresponsiveness**.

2. Shout for **help**.

3. Open the **airway**.

4. Look, listen, and feel for **breathing**.

5. Give 2 full **breaths**.

6. Check for a **pulse** at the side of the **neck**.

7. Have someone phone the **EMS system** for help.

8. Begin **rescue breathing**.

9. Give 1 breath every **5** seconds.

10. Keep the victim from moving until **EMS** personnel arrive, and keep checking the victim's **breathing** and **pulse**.

Review Question: First Aid for an Adult With an Obstructed Airway

You go into a restroom at a shopping mall and find someone lying on the floor. You survey the scene and see that it is safe to help. What would you do next?

Do a primary survey to check the ABCs.

1. Check for _consciousness_. (See clue below.)

2. Shout for _help_.

3. Position the _victim_.

4. Open the _airway_.

5. Look, listen, and feel for _breath_. (See clue.)

6. Give _two_ _full_ _breaths_. (See clue.)

7. _Retilt_ the head.

8. Give _2 full_ _breaths_ again. (See clue.)

9. Have someone phone the _EMS_ _service_ for help.

10. Give _6_ to _10_ abdominal thrusts. (See clue.)

11. Do a _finger_ _sweep_. (See clue.)

12. Open the airway and give 2 _full_ _breaths_. (See clue.)

13. Keep the victim from moving until _EMS_ personnel arrive, and keep checking the victim's _breathing_ and _pulse_.

CLUES:
- At step 1, the victim is unconscious.
- At step 5, the victim is not breathing.
- At step 6, you are unable to breathe air into the victim.
- At step 8, you are still unable to breathe air into the victim.
- At step 10, you hear a gasp coming from the victim's mouth during the sixth thrust. You immediately stop giving thrusts.
- At step 11, you find and remove a piece of food.
- After step 12, victim begins breathing on his own.

Answers

1. Check for **unresponsiveness**.

2. Shout for **help**.

3. Position the **victim**.

4. Open the **airway**.

5. Look, listen, and feel for **breathing**.

6. Give **2 full breaths**.

7. **Retilt** the head.

8. Give **2 full breaths** again.

9. Have someone phone the **EMS system** for help.

10. Give **6** to **10** abdominal thrusts.

11. Do a **finger sweep**.

12. Open the airway and give 2 **full breaths**.

13. Keep the victim from moving until **EMS** personnel arrive, and keep checking the victim's **breathing** and **pulse**.

Review Question: Recognizing the Signals of a Heart Attack

You are at a movie theater with your cousin and his wife. On the way out of the theater, your cousin stops and clutches his chest as if he is in great pain. When you ask him about it, he says he's fine, it's "just a little heartburn or indigestion." He is sweating and just doesn't look right. What do you do next?

1. Recognize the signals of a ___heart___ ___attack___.

2. Make your cousin ___sit___ or ___lie___ down in a comfortable position.

3. Have someone phone the ___EMS___ system for help.

   NO CLUES NEEDED

Answers

1. Recognize the signals of a **heart attack**.

2. Make your cousin **sit** or **lie** down in a comfortable position.

3. Have someone phone the **EMS** system for help.

Review Question: CPR for an Adult

You come to work early and find your boss lying facedown on the floor in the office. She is not moving, and there is no one else around. You survey the scene and see that it is safe to help her. What would you do next?

Do a primary survey to check the ABCs.

1. Check for _consciousness_. (See clue below.)

2. Shout for _help_.

3. Position the _victim_.

4. Open the _airway_.

5. Look, listen, and feel for _breath_. (See clue.)

6. Give 2 full _breaths_.

7. Check the carotid _pulse_. (See clue.)

8. Have someone phone the _EMS_ _system_ for help.

9. Give CPR: cycles of _15_ chest compressions and _2_ rescue breaths.

10. After 4 cycles of CPR, check the carotid _pulse_. (See clue.)

11. Give _2 full_ breaths.

12. Continue CPR until _EMS_ personnel arrive and take over.

   CLUES: • At step 1, the victim is unconscious.
   • At step 5, the victim is not breathing.
   • At step 7, the victim has no pulse.
   • At step 10, the victim still has no pulse.

Answers

1. Check for **unresponsiveness**.

2. Shout for **help**.

3. Position the **victim**.

4. Open the **airway**.

5. Look, listen, and feel for **breathing**.

6. Give 2 full **breaths**.

7. Check the carotid **pulse**.

8. Have someone phone the **EMS system** for help.

9. Give CPR: cycles of **15** chest compressions and **2** rescue breaths.

10. After 4 cycles of CPR, check the carotid **pulse**.

11. Give **2** breaths.

12. Continue CPR until **EMS** personnel arrive and take over.

Unit Two: Lifesaving Skills to Help Children and Infants

How Much Do You Know About Childhood Emergencies?

Here are some questions about respiratory and cardiac emergencies in children and infants. These questions should help you think about your role in dealing with and preventing such emergencies. Check the best answers. Do not feel disappointed if you are not able to answer every question correctly.

1. What is the leading cause of death in children ages one through 14 in the United States?
   ☐ Injury from accidents is the leading cause of death in children ages one through 14.
   ☐ Diseases such as measles, pneumonia, and chicken pox are the leading cause of death in children ages one through 14.
   ☐ Cardiovascular disease is the leading cause of death in children ages one through 14.

2. What is the safest way for an infant or toddler to ride in an automobile?
   ☐ The safest way for an infant or toddler to ride in an automobile is held in a passenger's arms.
   ☐ The safest way for an infant or toddler to ride in an automobile is buckled into an adult seat belt.
   ☐ The safest way for an infant or toddler to ride in an automobile is buckled into an approved car safety seat.

3. If an infant chokes on a piece of food and cannot cough, cry, or breathe, what should you do?
   ☐ You should give the infant a drink of water.
   ☐ You should give back blows followed by chest thrusts.
   ☐ You should hold the infant upside down by the ankles and shake the infant.

4. You are shopping in a supermarket when you hear a yell for help. You see a mother with a child in a cart. The child is coughing weakly. The mother says that the child is choking on a piece of candy. What would a trained person do?
   ☐ A trained person would run to get help.
   ☐ A trained person would give the child abdominal thrusts.
   ☐ A trained person would hold the child upside down by the ankles and shake the child.

Answers

1. **Injury from accidents is the leading cause of death in children ages one through 14.** A child is much more likely to die from an injury than from a disease. In Chapter 6, you will read about the most common injuries to children and infants. You will learn about ways to prevent these injuries.

2. **The safest way for an infant or toddler to ride in an automobile is buckled into an approved car safety seat.** A car safety seat will hold an infant or toddler securely and will help absorb the forces of even violent crashes.

3. If an infant chokes on a piece of food and cannot cough, cry, or breathe, **you should give back blows followed by chest thrusts.** In Chapter 11, you will learn first aid for an infant who is choking.

4. **A trained person would give the child abdominal thrusts.** You give abdominal thrusts to a conscious child who is choking. You will learn how to give abdominal thrusts in Chapter 8.

What Unit Two Will Teach You

Why Talk About Preventing Childhood Injuries

Each year millions of children in the United States under 15 years of age need medical care for injuries received as a result of accidents. Thousands of children in the United States are killed as a result of accidents. This is an important national problem.

For children ages one through 14, the leading cause of death is injury from accidents. For infants under one year old, injury from accidents is the fourth leading cause of death.

How to Reduce Childhood Injuries

To prevent accidental deaths and injuries to children and infants, you must know what factors increase their risk of being injured. You also must act to reduce the risk of injury. Chapter 6 will help you learn what you can do to protect infants and children. You will read about steps you can take to make a safer environment for children.

What You Can Do

If an illness or an accident causes a respiratory or cardiac emergency in a child or an infant, the correct first aid must be given immediately to save the child's or infant's life. You could be the person who gives that child a better chance of survival. This unit will tell you how to prevent and recognize certain conditions that may lead to respiratory or cardiac emergencies. The unit discusses when to begin emergency care and how to provide this care.

Children's hearts are usually healthy. Unlike adults, children do not often initially suffer a cardiac emergency. In most cases, the child first suffers a respiratory emergency that quite often goes unrecognized. Then a cardiac emergency develops. For this reason, it is important to learn how to prevent and recognize conditions that may lead to a respiratory or cardiac emergency.

The most common cause of respiratory and cardiac emergencies in children is injury from accidents. Motor vehicle accidents are the leading cause of injury. Other injuries that can cause respiratory and cardiac emergencies include those that result from near-drowning, smoke inhalation, burns, poisoning, airway obstruction, firearms, and falls.

Injuries, for example those resulting from a motor vehicle accident, can cause severe blood loss. Severe blood loss leads to shock. Signs of shock include agitation, drowsiness, change in skin color (to pale, blue, or gray), cool and/or moist skin, and increased heart rate. It is important to recognize the signals of shock because if untreated, shock may lead to a respiratory or cardiac emergency.

Respiratory and cardiac emergencies are also the result of foreign-body obstruction, medical conditions, and illness such as severe asthma, severe croup, and respiratory infections such as epiglottitis and bronchiolitis.

You have learned first aid for respiratory and cardiac emergencies in adults. In this unit, you will learn the early signals of respiratory and cardiac emergencies in children and infants. You will learn what to do when a child age one through eight or an infant newborn to age one has a respiratory or cardiac emergency. This unit will also give you information on how to prevent childhood injuries.

Objectives

By the time you finish reading this unit, you should be able to do the following:

1. *Describe ways to prevent childhood injuries and deaths.*
2. *Recognize respiratory and cardiac emergencies in children and infants.*
3. *Describe how to give first aid for respiratory and cardiac emergencies in children and infants.*

It is very important to be able to recognize the early signals of a respiratory emergency. These signals show that there is the potential for a life-threatening emergency. Signs of respiratory difficulty may include agitation, drowsiness, change in skin color (to pale, blue, or gray), increased difficulty in breathing, and increased heart and breathing rates.

If an infant or child displays any of these signs, you should begin emergency care and contact your emergency medical services (EMS) system immediately. This unit will help you learn how to give the correct first aid.

Another cause of cardiac emergencies is sudden infant death syndrome (SIDS). SIDS is a sudden event that is not typically preceded by respiratory difficulty. Thus, it cannot be predicted or recognized before a cardiac arrest occurs.

Research on SIDS suggests that—

- 90 percent of SIDS deaths occur while the infant is asleep (between midnight and 8 a.m.).
- SIDS deaths can occur between the ages of two weeks and 18 months, with the majority of deaths occurring between one and six months.
- The majority of SIDS deaths occur in fall and winter.
- 30 to 50 percent of SIDS victims have minor respiratory infections at the time of death.
- SIDS occurs slightly more often in males than in females.

If you discover an infant or child without a pulse, you should begin CPR and contact your EMS system immediately. You will learn how to give CPR to a child in Chapter 9 of this workbook and to an infant in Chapter 12.

Most emergency situations in which a child or infant requires CPR are preventable. As you read this workbook, think about what you can do to keep life-threatening emergencies from happening.

6

What You Can Do to Prevent Childhood Injuries

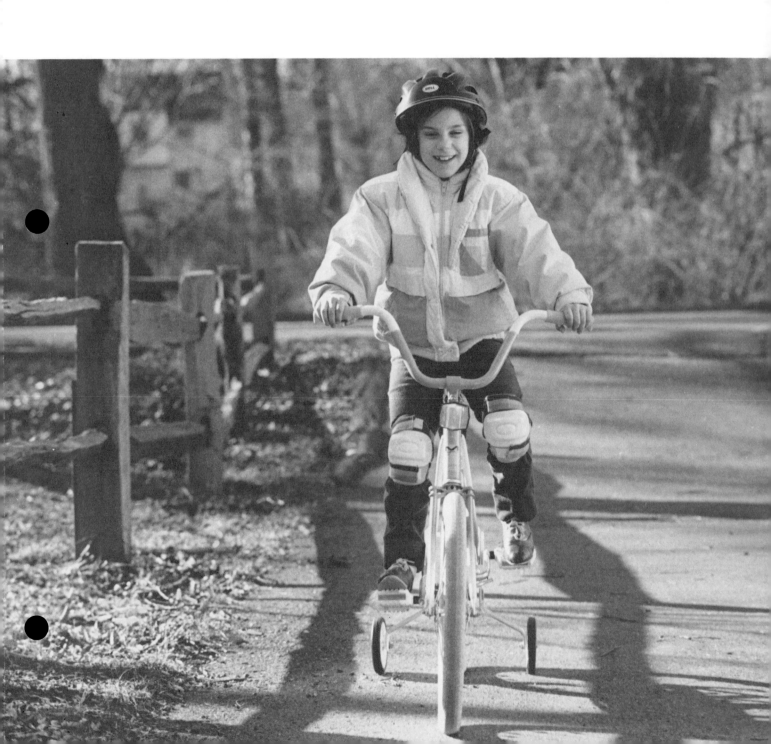

Parents do many things to keep their children healthy, like giving them good foods and taking them for checkups. Parents try to keep their children from getting sick. Children are given shots to prevent measles, mumps, and other diseases. But in the United States the greatest threat to the health of young children is not sickness. Each year about 8,300 children die from injuries resulting from accidents. Thousands more children are treated in hospitals for injuries. Many of these deaths and injuries could be prevented. This chapter will help you learn specific steps you can take to help prevent injury to children.

Objectives

By the time you finish reading this chapter, you should be able to do the following:

1. Identify the major causes of injuries to infants and children.
2. List the three basic parts of an injury-prevention plan.
3. Describe injury-prevention plans for children of different ages and stages of development.

Becoming Safety Conscious

There are three ways that you can help prevent injuries to children. One is to keep children away from things that might harm them. For example, don't let a child play with a carving knife. The second way is to stay near children so that you can act in case of danger. For example, if you are bathing a toddler, stay beside the tub so you can catch the child in case of a fall. The third way is to follow safety rules yourself and teach them to children. For example, cross streets with a green light or walk signal, and teach children to wait for the green light and look for cars before crossing.

Later in this chapter, you will learn how to develop a specific plan to prevent injuries to your own children, if you are a parent, or to other children that you take care of. But first, think about some general safety rules. These rules suggest some things you can do to protect children of all ages. Later you will read about safety rules for children in specific age groups.

General Safety Rules

Here are some safety rules you should follow to protect children:

1. Think ahead, anticipate danger.
2. Always expect children to be curious.
3. "Buckle up" children in motor vehicles.
4. Always supervise children in or near water.
5. Check your home for fire and burn dangers.
6. Be prepared for an emergency.

Let's take a closer look at these rules to see what they mean.

1. **Think ahead, anticipate danger.**

   Try to think about how injuries might happen. A child who is riding a bicycle, for example, might fall off or be hit by a car. Once you are aware of dangers, you can take steps to prevent injuries. For example, you could buy the child a helmet for head protection. Making sure the bicycle is the correct size and has no broken parts can reduce the chance of injury *(Fig. 45)*. Becoming safety conscious is an important part of preventing injuries.

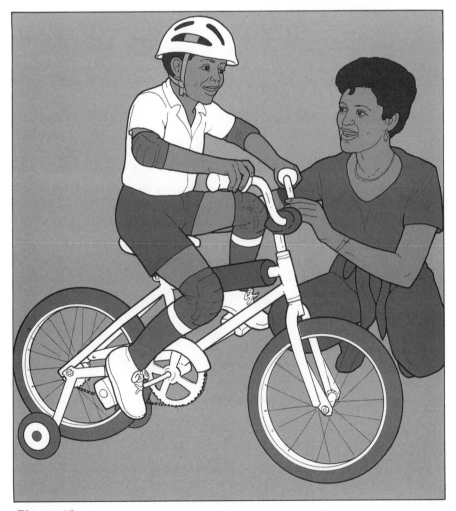

Figure 45
Think Ahead to Prevent Injuries

2. **Always expect children to be curious.**

   Children are explorers by nature. Their curiosity leads them to touch, taste, poke, pull, reach, and climb. As they grow and develop new skills, their curiosity can lead them into danger. What you do to protect them from injury must allow for their curiosity and their ever-changing skills.

3. **"Buckle up" children in motor vehicles.**

   Infants and young children should always be buckled into approved car safety seats *(Fig. 46)*. They should never ride in a passenger's arms. Always install and use a car safety seat correctly, following the manufacturer's directions. As the child grows, the type of restraint will change, from a car safety seat, to a booster seat, to adult safety belts. The important thing is that children should always be in seats and/or belts suitable for their age.

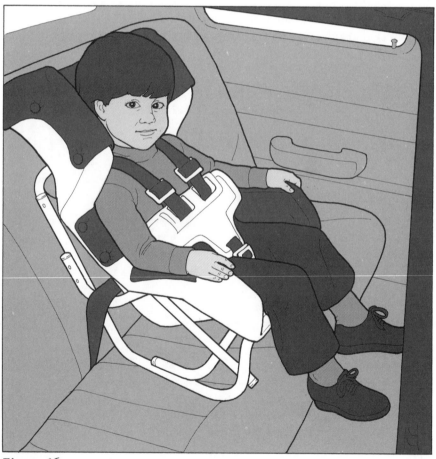

Figure 46
"Buckle up" Children in Motor Vehicles

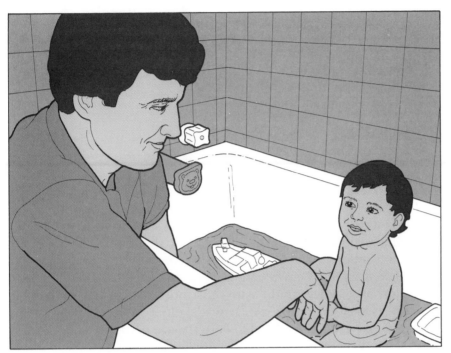

Figure 47
Always Supervise Children in Water

4. **Always supervise children in or near water.**
   Young children can drown in as little as two inches of water.
   Never leave them alone either in or near a bathtub, wading or
   swimming pool, pond, etc. ***(Fig. 47)***.

5. **Check your home for fire and burn dangers.**
   Take steps to prevent fires, for example by making sure that the
   electrical wiring in your home meets safety codes. Install smoke
   detectors to warn you in case of fire. Check smoke detectors often
   to make sure that they are working. To reduce the risk of tapwater
   burns, turn your hot water heater to 120° F.

6. **Be prepared for an emergency.**
   Place fire extinguishers in your home where a fire is most likely to
   happen, such as the kitchen. Make a plan so family members can
   escape in case of fire, and practice your plan. Take a Red Cross
   first aid course.
      Prepare for poisoning emergencies by buying syrup of ipecac at
   a drug store. Syrup of ipecac is used in some cases of poisoning to
   make a child vomit. If you suspect that a child has had contact
   with a poison, telephone your area Poison Control Center.

Post a list of emergency numbers by each telephone in the home. This list should include the following numbers:

- Emergency medical services (EMS) system
- Fire Department
- Police Department
- Poison Control Center
- Parents' work
- Physician
- Close neighbor

Making a Child's World Safer

Making safer places for children to explore and play in is an important part of preventing injury. General safety rules give some guidelines, but there are many very specific things that you can do to safeguard children. These specific actions must be related to a child's age. Making a child's environment safe is not something that can be done just once. Since children are constantly learning new skills, their caregivers must constantly take new and different precautions. These precautions have to be related to both the age of the child and the child's skills and activities.

This chapter deals with three age groups:

- Infants—from birth to age one
- Toddlers and preschoolers—ages one to five
- Young school-age children—ages five to nine

Each age group has its special needs, because as children grow, they rapidly develop new skills. The interests and activities of each age group also differ from those of other age groups.

Developing an Injury-Prevention Plan

If you want to help prevent injuries to children, you need to develop a personal plan. Make safety plans according to the age of the child you want to protect. The plan must be very specific. To help you develop a personal plan, the rest of this chapter presents brief descriptions of the three age groups: infants, toddlers and pre-schoolers, and young school-age children. An injury-prevention plan is suggested for each of the three age groups.

Each injury-prevention plan is divided into three parts as follows:

1. **Remove dangers**.

   A dangerous situation creates a risk of injury. For example, a bottle of poisonous furniture polish stored under a kitchen sink is a danger to a toddler. It is possible that the child will drink the polish and be poisoned. The danger can easily be removed by storing the polish where the child cannot reach it.

2. Give supervision.

Supervision means watching over a child and knowing what the child is doing all the time. This means that you are always with the child or nearby, or someone else has this responsibility. Children are often injured when they are left alone and unsupervised for even a few minutes. Supervision is an important part of keeping a child safe. The amount of supervision needed changes as a child grows and develops.

3. Teach safety.

You can teach safety in two ways. First, you can set an example of safe behavior by acting safely yourself. Second, you can encourage children to act safely, showing them what they **should do,** for example, buckle their seat belts. You should also teach them what they **should not do,** for example, touch a hot stove. But remember, it takes time to learn safe behavior and to make it a habit.

Review Questions

Fill in the blanks with the right word.

1. The three basic parts of an injury-prevention plan for children are—
   a. Remove _danger_.
   b. Give _supervision_.
   c. Teach _safety_.

2. Six general safety rules to prevent injuries to children of all ages are—
   a. _Plan_ ahead, anticipate danger.
   b. Expect children to be _curious_.
   c. "_Buckle_ _up_" children in motor vehicles.
   d. _Supervise_ children in or near water.
   e. Check your home for fire and _burn_ dangers.
   f. Be _prepared_ for an emergency.

Answers

1. The three basic parts of an injury-prevention plan for children are—
   a. Remove **dangers**.
   b. Give **supervision**.
   c. Teach **safety**.

2. Six general safety rules to prevent injuries to children of all ages are—
   a. **Think** ahead, anticipate danger.
   b. Expect children to be **curious**.
   c. **"Buckle up"** children in motor vehicles.
   d. **Supervise** children in or near water.
   e. Check your home for fire and **burn** dangers.
   f. Be **prepared** for an emergency.

Preventing Injuries to Infants

About Infants

When infants are born, they are dependent on their parents and other adults. But from birth, infants learn how to control their body. Newborn infants squirm and wave their arms and legs. Soon they learn to lift their head, roll over, and grasp things. Later they learn how to sit, crawl, and stand. With each new skill, they can learn more by moving and touching, hearing, seeing, and tasting.

Curious infants learn about their world by putting objects in their mouth. They grasp and pull with their hands. Their curiosity can lead them into danger. The infant who can wiggle can roll off a bed and break a leg. The infant who can grasp buttons, beads, or other small objects can put them in his or her mouth and choke. The infant who can pull things from a table can be burned by a hot cup of coffee. As infants grow, they face new dangers as they learn to roll, creep and crawl, stand, climb, and walk. But they cannot recognize danger, and it is up to adults to protect them.

Some of the steps that parents and other caregivers can take to prevent injuries to infants are shown in the chart, "What You Can Do to Prevent Injuries to Infants." As you read this chart, keep in mind that for infants motor vehicle accidents are the leading cause of death due to injuries. Other common injuries are choking, suffocation, burns and injuries from house fires, near-drowning, falls, and poisoning.

The chart shows you some of the actions you can take to reduce the risks of injury and death in infants. Use the chart to make your own three-part injury-prevention plan.

Injury Risks	Prevention Steps
Car-related	**1. Remove Dangers** Buckle infants into car safety seat on each and every ride. Use only an approved car safety seat. Install the safety seat correctly. The seat should face the rear of the car until the infant weighs about 20 pounds.
Choking	Don't leave small objects (buttons, coins, beads, small pieces of older children's toys, etc.) within an infant's reach. Check infants' toys to make sure they are too large to be swallowed and have no small, detachable parts like buttons. Give infants soft food that does not require chewing. Cut food for older infants into small pieces, especially food like hot dogs. Do not give infants nuts, raw vegetables, popcorn, etc.
Suffocation/ Strangulation	Keep plastic bags and filmy plastic away from infants. Use a crib with slats 2⅜ inches apart or less and a snug-fitting mattress. Keep furniture such as cribs, play pens, and high chairs away from drapery cords and electric appliance cords. Never hang rattles, pacifiers, or other objects around an infant's neck. If an infant can sit up, don't hang toys across the crib.
Burns and House Fires	Check your home for fire hazards. (Ask your local fire department for help with this.) Set the thermostat on your water heater to 120°F. Install smoke detectors and keep them in working order by testing them and replacing batteries when needed. Check the bathwater temperature to make sure it is not too hot. Do not cook while holding an infant. Keep hot foods and liquids and lit cigarettes out of an infant's reach. Keep handles on pots and pans turned to the back of the stove when you cook. Put barriers around fireplaces, radiators, hot pipes, wood-burning stoves, and other hot surfaces to separate infants from them. Place high chairs away from stoves. Make sure the electric cords of irons, coffee makers, and other hot appliances are not hanging from counters. Put safety covers or tape on electric outlets. Buy flame-resistant clothing, especially sleepwear
Falls	Stay with an infant who is on a bed or changing table. Put barriers at the top and bottom of stairs before an infant begins to creep and crawl.

What You Can Do to Prevent Injuries to Infants

Injury Risks	Prevention Steps
Falls (*continued*)	Hold the handrail when you carry an infant down the stairs.
	Use skidproof mats or stickers in the bathtub.
	Keep stairways clear of objects that could cause you to fall while holding an infant.
	Choose a high chair that is stable and wide-based and that has a seat belt.
	Be sure all low windows are locked and well screened.
Poisoning	Use nontoxic finishes and lead-free paint when painting and refinishing toys and infants' furniture.
	Store all prescription and nonprescription medicines in locked cupboards.
	Keep all medicines in original containers.
	Store alcohol in locked cabinets.
	Keep house plants out of reach.
	See that all handbags, including those of visiting friends and relatives, are out of reach.
	Buy a bottle of syrup of ipecac to be used as directed in case of poisoning.
	Keep cleaning supplies in original containers and store them out of reach.
	Keep cosmetics such as nail polish and hair spray out of reach.
	Store basement and garage supplies such as moth balls, paints, and fertilizers out of reach.
	2. Give Supervision
Drowning (both indoors and outdoors)	Stay with infants while they are in or near water, whether in the tub or in a wading or swimming pool.
Falls	Do not leave an infant in an infant seat alone when the infant seat is on a table or counter.
	Stay with an infant on a bed or changing table.
Choking	Never leave a bottle propped up for an infant to drink unsupervised.
General	**3. Teach Safety** Use your tone of voice and simple phrases such as "No, don't touch" and "Not for baby" as a start to safety education for your infant.
	Behave safely yourself.

Review Questions

3. Which injuries are among the most common in infants?
   (Check four.)
   - ☑ a. Injuries from motor vehicle accidents
   - ☑ b. Choking
   - ☑ c. Injuries from fires and burns
   - ☑ d. Drowning
   - ☐ e. Animal bites

4. Which of the following are generally true of infants?
   (Check all that apply.)
   - ☐ a. They are able to recognize danger.
   - ☑ b. They are curious.
   - ☑ c. They put objects in their mouth.
   - ☑ d. They are constantly learning.

5. Which of the following steps will help prevent choking injuries in
   infants? (Check all that apply.)
   - ☑ a. Removing small objects from an infant's reach
   - ☐ b. Putting barriers at the top and bottom of stairs
   - ☑ c. Feeding an infant soft foods that don't require chewing
   - ☐ d. Keeping hot liquids out of an infant's reach

Answers

3. These are among the most common injuries in infants:
   a. **Injuries from motor vehicle accidents**
   b. **Choking**
   c. **Injuries from fires and burns**
   d. **Drowning**

4. The following are generally true of infants:
   b. **They are curious.**
   c. **They put objects in their mouth.**
   d. **They are constantly learning.**

5. The following steps will help prevent choking injuries in infants:
   a. **Removing small objects from an infant's reach**
   c. **Feeding an infant soft foods that don't require chewing**

Preventing Injuries to Toddlers and Preschoolers

About Toddlers and Preschoolers

Like infants, toddlers and preschoolers are constantly exploring and trying new things. However, in other ways toddlers and preschoolers are very different from infants. They can walk and do more with their body than infants can. They can use words to ask for things and talk to other people.

Toddlers and preschoolers have learned a lot, but they are still very different from adults. For example, toddlers do not realize that what happens to them in one situation might happen to them in another, similar situation. They do not understand cause and effect. A toddler who falls off a fence once will probably continue to climb and fall. The child is not able to think, "If I climb that fence, I might fall and hurt myself." For this reason, supervision is important. Toddlers and preschoolers need simple, clear instructions: "Don't climb the fence." They also need to be reminded often about what they should and should not do.

Some of the steps that parents and other caregivers can take to prevent injuries to toddlers and preschoolers are shown in the chart, "What You Can Do to Prevent Injuries to Toddlers and Preschoolers." As you read this chart, keep in mind that motor vehicle accidents are the leading cause of injury and death to children in this age group. Other common injuries are near-drowning, burns and injuries from house fires, choking, falls, and poisoning. The chart shows you some of the actions you can take to reduce the risk of injuries to toddlers and preschoolers. Use the chart to make your own three-part injury-prevention plan.

What You Can Do to Prevent Injuries to Toddlers and Preschoolers

Injury Risks	Prevention Steps
Car-related	**1. Remove Dangers** Buckle toddlers and preschoolers into approved car safety seats on each and every ride. Use only an approved car safety seat. Install the safety seat correctly. Make sure toddlers and preschoolers play in areas separated from traffic.
Burns and House Fires	Check your home for fire dangers. (Ask your fire department for help with this.) Set thermostat on water heater to 120°F. Install smoke detectors and keep them in working order by testing them and replacing batteries when needed. Check bathwater temperature to make sure it is not too hot. Keep electric cords out of toddlers' and preschoolers' reach. Keep toddlers and preschoolers away from the stove, iron, and other dangerous appliances. Put outlet covers on electric outlets, and move furniture so that outlets are not easily seen or touched. Keep hot foods and liquids and lit cigarettes out of reach. Keep matches, lighters, and cigarettes out of small children's sight and reach. Put barriers around fireplaces, radiators, hot pipes, and other hot surfaces to separate children from them. Buy flame-resistant clothing, especially sleepwear.
Choking	Choose toys that are too large to be swallowed and that have no small, detachable parts. Do not give toddlers and preschoolers nuts, popcorn, raw vegetables, and other foods that could cause choking. Cut foods such as hot dogs into small pieces. Seat toddlers and preschoolers in a high chair or at a table for meals and snacks.
Falls	Check to be sure playground equipment is in good condition. Sand or cedar chips under play equipment make it safer. Put barriers at the top and bottom of stairs until toddlers show that they are steady on their feet and can use handrails properly. Make household rugs skidproof. Use skidproof mats or stickers in the bathtub. Don't give children toys with sharp edges or points.

What You Can Do to Prevent Injuries to Toddlers and Preschoolers

Injury Risks	Prevention Steps
Falls *(continued)*	Cushion sharp edges of furniture with cotton and masking tape or commercial corner guards. Keep doors to porches, attics, laundry rooms, and basements locked. Put window guards in rooms above the first floor. Be sure all low windows are locked and well screened. Lock the sides of a crib at the highest level and put the mattress at the lowest level to prevent a child from climbing out.
Poisoning	Keep all medicines in original containers. Store all medicines in a locked cabinet, your shoulder height or higher. Keep house plants out of reach. Buy a bottle of syrup of ipecac to be used as directed in case of poisoning. Store alcohol in locked cabinets. Keep cosmetics, such as nail polish and hair spray, out of reach. Keep cleaning supplies in original containers and store them out of reach and out of sight. Store basement and garage supplies such as moth balls, paints, and fertilizers out of reach. See that all handbags are out of reach. Always use nontoxic finishes and lead-free paint on toys and furniture.
Drowning	If you have a home swimming pool, fence it completely around to prevent access from the house by your child.
Drowning (both indoors and outdoors)	**2. Give Supervision** Stay with toddlers and preschoolers when they are in or near water, whether in the tub or in a pool. Schedule baths at times when adults (rather than older children) can supervise.
Falls	Seat children in a high chair for snacks and meals, and use a seat belt. Supervise children so that they do not climb out of or fall from the high chair. Supervise climbing activity. Supervise both outdoor and indoor play.
Car-related	**3. Teach Safety** Be a positive role model by "buckling up" yourself and talking about what you are doing.

What You Can Do to Prevent Injuries to Toddlers and Preschoolers

Injury Risks	Prevention Steps
Burns and House Fires	Teach toddlers the meaning of "hot."
	Teach preschoolers to give matches they find to grown-ups.
	Teach preschoolers what to do if their clothing catches fire.
Poisoning	Teach toddlers and preschoolers not to eat any parts of indoor or outdoor plants, unless you say it is okay.
General	Give specific safety instructions: "Don't climb the tree." "Stay inside the fence."
	Frequently remind toddlers and preschoolers what they should and should not do.
	Teach toddlers to respond to words like "stop" and "no" that you can use in case of danger.
	Teach preschoolers to tell an adult if they (or anyone else) are hurt.
Medical Identification Bracelet	A child with a special medical problem should always wear an identification bracelet.

Review Questions

6. Which injuries are among the most common in toddlers and preschoolers? (Check all that apply.)
   - ☑ a. Injuries from motor vehicle accidents
   - ☑ b. Near-drowning
   - ☑ c. Burns
   - ☑ d. Choking
   - ☐ e. Injuries from firearms

7. Which of the following statements describe toddlers or preschoolers? (Check all that apply.)
   - ☑ a. They are constantly trying new things.
   - ☑ b. They frequently fall.
   - ☐ c. They understand cause and effect.
   - ☑ d. They need to be reminded often about what they should and should not do.

8. Suppose the following situations exist in a toddler's home. Which are dangers that should be removed to prevent injury to the toddler? (Check all that apply.)
   - ☑ a. The hot water temperature is set at 145° F.
   - ☐ b. Fireplace has a screen.
   - ☑ c. Matches are kept on the coffee table.
   - ☐ d. Outlet covers are on unused electrical outlets.

Answers

6. The following are among the most common injuries in toddlers and preschoolers:
   a. **Injuries from motor vehicle accidents**
   b. **Near-drowning**
   c. **Burns**
   d. **Choking**

7. The following statements describe toddlers or preschoolers:
   a. **They are constantly trying new things.**
   b. **They frequently fall.**
   d. **They need to be reminded often about what they should and should not do.**

8. These are dangers that should be removed to prevent injury to a toddler:
   a. **The hot water temperature is set at 145° F.** (The thermostat should be set at 120° F.)
   c. **Matches are kept on the coffee table.**
   (Matches should be kept where a toddler cannot reach them.)

Preventing Injuries to Young School-Age Children

About Young School-Age Children

The world of children five to nine years old includes the school and neighborhood as well as the home. Young school-age children spend a lot of time away from their parents. Playing with other children is very important. Learning new skills—like riding a bicycle or scooter—is also important. These children want to show their parents, their friends, and themselves just how much they can do. Although they might "know the rules," they are likely to test them. This is normal for children as they grow and try to find out more about themselves and the world around them.

During the years from five to nine, children grow quickly and learn so many new skills that it may be difficult for adults to judge their abilities correctly. In making safety rules, adults have to remember that children still think differently from adults. For example, children frequently misjudge how far away a car is and how fast it is going. They sometimes mix up left and right and do not understand many traffic signs. Thus, it may be difficult for them to cross a street or ride a bicycle in the street safely.

Some of the steps that parents and other caregivers can take to prevent injuries to young school-age children are shown in the chart, "What You Can Do to Prevent Injuries to Young School-Age Children." As you read this chart, keep in mind that motor vehicle accidents are the leading cause of injuries and death for this age group. Other common injuries result from bicycles and other riding equipment, near-drowning, falls, and sports activities.

The chart shows you some of the actions you can take to reduce the risk of injury and death to young school-age children. Use the chart to develop your own three-part injury-prevention plan.

What You Can Do to Prevent Injuries to Young School-Age Children

Injury Risks	Prevention Steps
Car-related (passenger and pedestrian)	**1. Remove Dangers** Be sure that children "buckle up" properly for each and every ride. Make sure that children play in areas separated from traffic.
Burns and House Fires	Check your home for fire hazards. (Ask your fire department for help with this.) Install smoke detectors and keep them in working order by testing them and replacing batteries when needed. Set the thermostat on your water heater to 120°F. Keep matches, lighters, and cigarettes out of reach. Buy flame-resistant clothing, especially sleepwear.
Bicycles	Check children's bicycles to make sure the size is appropriate. Be sure that bicycles, scooters, and other riding toys do not have any broken parts. Buy an approved helmet for the child to wear when riding and teach him or her to put it on correctly.
Falls	Check playgrounds to make sure the equipment is in good condition. Soft sand or cedar chips under play equipment make it safer.
Drowning	If you have a home swimming pool, fence it completely around to prevent access from the house by your child.
Bicycles	**2. Give Supervision** Make sure that a child wears a helmet when riding a bicycle.
Drowning	Supervise children's water play.
General	Since you are not always with your children, be familiar with the places they usually go. For instance, you should be familiar with the route to school, the school yard, neighbors' houses, and where your children go after school. Be sure you know how other caregivers supervise your children when you are not there. Make clear the kind of supervision you expect for your children.
Car-related	**3. Teach Safety** Be a positive role model by always "buckling up" yourself.
Bicycles	Teach children safe riding practices such as obeying traffic signs. Stress the importance of not fooling around with other children while riding.

What You Can Do to Prevent Injuries to Young School-Age Children

Injury Risks	Prevention Steps
Sports-related	Teach children how to use sports equipment properly and to always wear the safety equipment needed for a sport.
Medical Information Bracelet	If a child has a special medical problem, he or she should wear an identification bracelet, and the school should know about this special situation.
Drowning	Teach children to swim. Teach water safety, and give specific rules for swimming, boating, etc.
Burns and House Fires	Teach children not to play with matches.
General	Teach children their telephone number, address, and parents' work telephone numbers. Make sure that young school-age children know how to call the emergency number for the EMS system, police, and fire department. Many communities use 911.
	Discuss safety rules covering your children's environment: in the house, in the yard, crossing the street, going to school.
	Reinforce the safety education your children's school provides.

Review Questions

9. Which statements describe a young school-age child?
   (Check all that apply.)
   ☒ a. Usually plays with children the same age
   ☐ b. Spends more time at home
   ☐ c. Always follows safety rules
   ☒ d. Wants to show how much he or she can do

10. Which of the following are good ways to teach safety to young school-age children?
    (Check all that apply.)
    ☐ a. Teach them safety rules for swimming, boating, etc.
    ☒ b. Teach them the emergency number in your community.
    ☒ c. Always wear your own seat belt in the car.
    ☒ d. Supervise children using playground equipment.

Answers

9. These statements describe a young school-age child:
   a. **Usually plays with children the same age**
   d. **Wants to show how much he or she can do**

10. These are good ways to teach safety to young school-age children:
    a. **Teach them safety rules for swimming, boating, etc.**
    b. **Teach them the emergency number in your community.**
    c. **Always wear your own seat belt in the car.**

One Last Word

This chapter has outlined ways you can prevent children's injuries. Children are routinely protected against measles, polio, and other diseases by being immunized. You can provide equally important protection by removing dangers, giving supervision, and teaching safety. You can reduce the risk of injuries by making safety an important part of the way you care for children.

A good way to start is by completing the Home Safety Checklist on pages 296 through 298 of this workbook. The checklist will help you identify dangers in your home so you can remove them.

Certainly, the world is full of risks for people of all ages. But by thinking ahead and taking preventive steps, you can greatly reduce risks to children.

7

What to Do When a Child's Breathing Stops (Rescue Breathing)

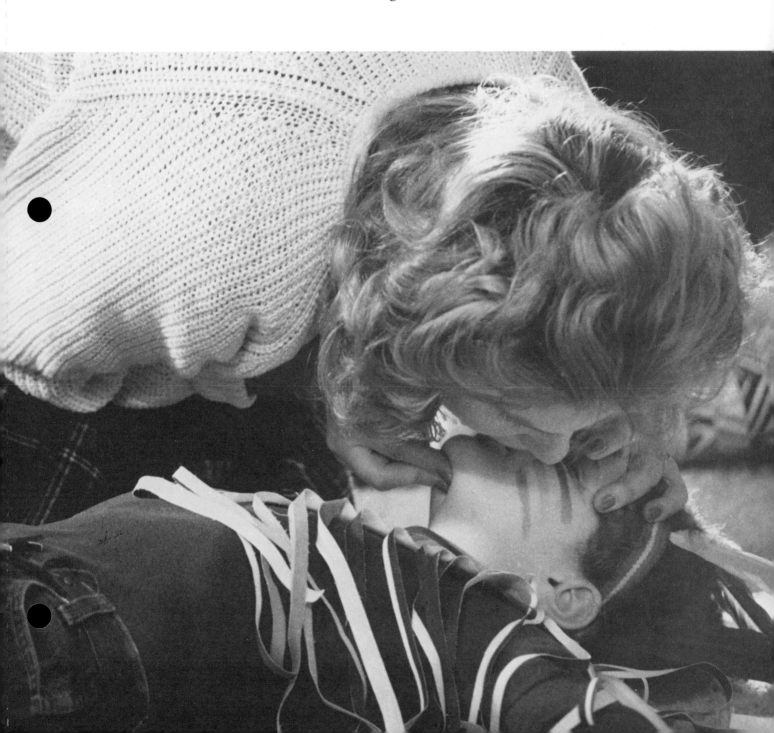

What to Do When a Child's Breathing Stops (Rescue Breathing)

Age 1 thru 8

In Chapter 2, you learned rescue breathing for an adult. To give rescue breathing to a child, you need to learn a different technique. In this chapter, you will learn rescue breathing for a child age one through eight.

Objectives

By the time you finish reading this chapter, you should be able to do the following:

1. Describe the early signals of a respiratory emergency.
2. Describe when a child needs rescue breathing.
3. Describe how to position a child for rescue breathing.
4. Describe how to give rescue breathing to a child.

Respiratory Emergencies in Children

Rescue breathing is given to a child whose breathing has stopped but whose heart is still beating. Injuries resulting from motor vehicle accidents, near-drowning, smoke inhalation, burns, poisoning, and airway obstruction can cause a respiratory emergency.

A respiratory emergency can also result from a medical condition or illness such as severe croup, severe asthma, or respiratory infections such as epiglottitis.

It is important to recognize the early signals of a respiratory emergency. These signals may include any of the following:

- Agitation
- Drowsiness
- Change in skin color (to pale, blue, or gray)
- Increased difficulty in breathing
- Increased heart and breathing rates

If a child displays any of these signs, you should begin first aid as described below. By recognizing a potential respiratory emergency and/or dealing with one when it occurs, you may prevent a cardiac emergency from happening.

How to Give Rescue Breathing to a Child

If you find a child lying on the ground and not moving, you should quickly survey the scene and do a primary survey.

1. **Check for Unresponsiveness**
   The first thing you should do is check to see if the child is conscious. Tap or gently shake the child's shoulder. Shout, "Are you OK?" *(Fig. 48)*.

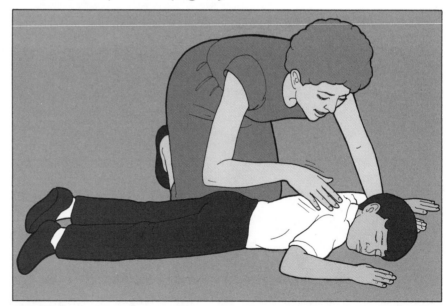

Figure 48
Check for Unresponsiveness

2. Shout for Help

If the child does not move or make a noise, shout for help.
Do this to get the attention of people you can ask to phone
the EMS system for help after you complete a primary survey
(Fig. 49).

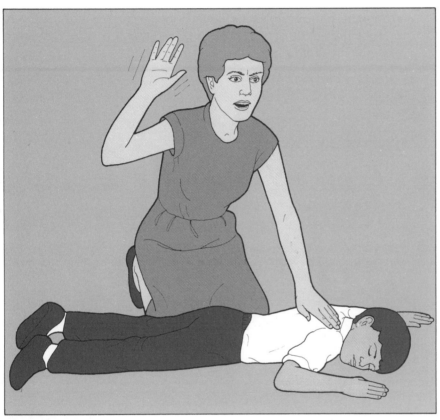

Figure 49
Shout for Help

3. **Position the Child**

   Move the child onto his or her back. To do this, roll the child as a unit *(Fig. 50)*. This will help to avoid twisting the body and making any injuries worse. To position the child—

   • Kneel facing the child, midway between the child's hips and shoulders.

   • Straighten the child's legs, if necessary.

   • Move the child's arm closest to you so that it is stretched out above the child's head.

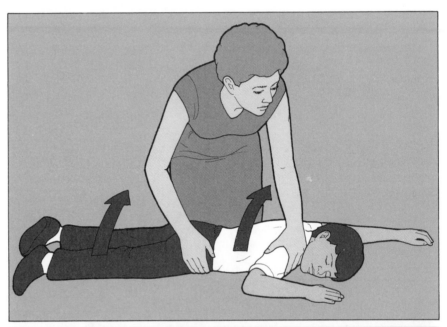

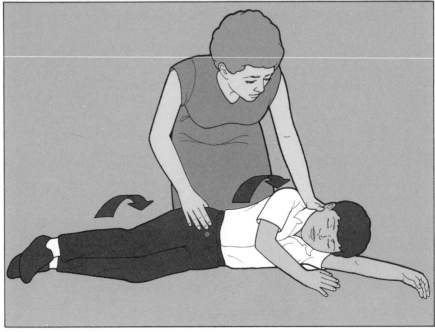

Figure 50
Position the Child

- Lean over the child and place one hand on the child's shoulder and the other on the child's hip.
- Roll the child toward you as a single unit by pulling slowly and evenly. Don't let the child's head and body twist.
- As you roll the child onto his or her back, move your hand from the shoulder to support the back of the head and neck.
- Place child's arm closest to you alongside the child's body.

It is important to position the child on his or her back as quickly as possible. It should take no more than 10 seconds to do this.

Note: Some children who require rescue breathing or CPR may have received a serious injury to the head, neck, or back. Moving these children, or opening the airway as described below, may result in further injury. Additional methods for handling these children are discussed in the American Red Cross CPR: Basic Life Support for the Professional Rescuer course.

4. **"A"—Open the Airway**

Immediately open the child's airway using the head-tilt/chin-lift *(Fig. 51)*. This is the most important action you can take to help the child survive. To open the airway—

- Kneel beside the child's head.
- Put your hand—the one nearest the child's head—on the child's forehead.
- Place one or two fingers (not the thumb) of your other hand under the bony part of the child's lower jaw at the chin.
- Tilt the child's head gently back by applying pressure on the forehead and lifting the chin. Don't close the child's mouth completely. Don't push in on the soft parts under the chin.

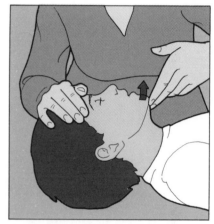

Figure 51
Head-Tilt/Chin-Lift

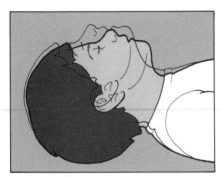

Figure 52
Range of Neutral-Plus Positions

Tilt the head gently back into the **neutral-plus** position. "Neutral-plus" is a term used to describe the amount of head-tilt necessary to open the airway of a child. Because a child's airway is different from that of an adult or an infant, and because a child's airway changes with age, there is more than one position for opening the airway. The term "neutral-plus" refers to a range of positions. This range is illustrated in *Figure 52*.

Begin by tilting the child's head into the neutral position. Remember to lift the chin. Check for breathlessness as described in step 5. Give 2 slow breaths, and watch for the chest to rise and fall as described in step 6. If the chest does not rise and fall, tilt the head slightly farther back and give 2 slow breaths. Again, watch for the chest to rise and fall.

If necessary, continue tilting the head slightly farther back, and continue giving rescue breaths until the chest rises and falls with each breath.

Once you have found the correct position, take note of it so you can place the child's head in this position each time you give breaths.

Remember: You will know that you have found the correct position when you see the child's chest rise and fall with each breath you give.

5. **"B"—Check for Breathlessness** (Look, listen, and feel for breathing.)
With the child's head in the neutral-plus position and the chin lifted, check to see if the child is breathing *(Fig. 53)*.
Tilting the head into the neutral-plus position and lifting the chin opens the airway and may in itself restore breathing. To check the child's breathing—
- Place your ear just over the child's mouth and nose and look at the child's chest.
- Look, listen, and feel. **Look** for the chest and abdomen to rise and fall, **listen** for breathing, and **feel** for air coming out of the child's nose and mouth. Do this for 3 to 5 seconds.

If the child is breathing, you will see the chest and abdomen move, and you will hear and feel air escaping at your ear and cheek. Movement of the chest and abdomen does not always mean that the child is breathing. He or she may be making unsuccessful attempts to breathe.

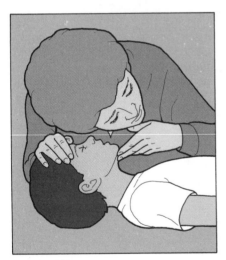

Figure 53
Check for Breathlessness

6. Give 2 Slow Breaths

If the child is not breathing, you must get air into the lungs at once *(Fig. 54)*. To give breaths—

- While keeping the airway open with the head-tilt/chin-lift, gently pinch the child's nose shut with the thumb and index finger of your hand that is on the child's forehead.
- Open your mouth wide. Take a breath. Seal your lips tightly around the outside of the child's mouth.
- Give 2 slow breaths at the rate of 1 to 1½ seconds per breath. Remove your mouth between breaths just long enough for you to take a breath. Watch for the chest to rise while you breathe into the child. Watch for the chest to fall after each breath. Listen and feel for air escaping as the child's chest falls.

If you feel resistance when you breathe into the child and air will not go in, the most likely cause is that you have not opened the airway properly. Retilt the child's head and give 2 slow breaths. If air still does not go into the child's lungs, the airway may be blocked by food or some other material. Chapter 8 describes how to help a child with an airway obstruction caused by food or another object.

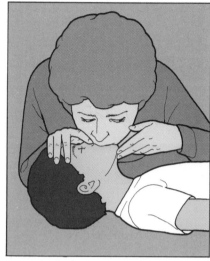

Figure 54
Mouth-to-Mouth Breathing

7. "C"—Check Circulation by Checking for a Pulse at the Side of the Neck

Check to see if the child's heart is beating by feeling for a pulse at the side of the neck. This pulse is called the **carotid pulse** *(Fig. 55)*. To check for a carotid pulse—

- Keep one hand on the child's forehead to keep the head in the neutral-plus position. Use your other hand—the one nearest the child's feet—to find the pulse. First, place your index and middle fingers on the child's Adam's apple. Then slide your fingers toward you into the groove between the windpipe and the muscle at the side of the neck. This is where you can feel the child's carotid pulse.
- Press gently with your fingertips to feel for the beat of the pulse. Be sure to feel for the pulse on the side of the neck closest to you. **Do not use your thumb** because you may feel your own pulse. Feel for the carotid pulse for 5 to 10 seconds.

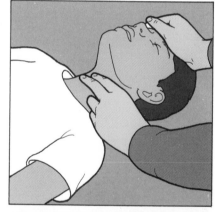

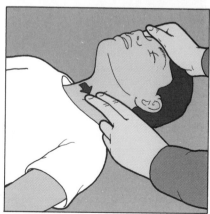

Figure 55
Locate and Feel Carotid Pulse

2 difference adult a child

neutral-plus position

1,2,3, breath

8. Phone the EMS System

After you have checked the pulse, you will have enough information about the child's condition to give to the bystanders you are sending to phone the EMS system. Tell the bystanders whether the child is conscious, breathing, and has a pulse. Tell them to give this information to the EMS dispatcher.

9. Begin Rescue Breathing

If you feel a pulse and the child is not breathing, then begin rescue breathing. (If you do not feel a pulse, the child's heart has stopped, and you must start CPR, which you will learn in Chapter 9.) To give rescue breathing—

- Keep the child's airway open using the head-tilt/chin-lift.
- Give 1 breath every 4 seconds. Take 1 to 1½ seconds to give each breath. A good way to do this is to count, "One one-thousand, two one-thousand, three one-thousand." Take a breath yourself and then breathe into the child. Look for the chest to rise as you breathe into the child.
- Between breaths, remove your mouth from the child. Look for the chest to fall as you listen and feel at the child's mouth and nose for escaping air. Listen to hear if the child starts breathing again.

10. Recheck Pulse

After 1 minute of rescue breathing (about 15 breaths), you should check the child's pulse. To check the pulse—

- Keep the airway open with the hand on the child's forehead.
- With your other hand feel for the carotid pulse for 5 seconds. If the child has a pulse, then check for breathing for 3 to 5 seconds. If the child is breathing, keep the airway open and monitor breathing and pulse closely. This means that you should look, listen, and feel for breathing and keep checking the pulse once every minute. Cover the child, and keep the child warm and as quiet as possible.

If the child is not breathing, continue rescue breathing and keep checking the pulse once every minute. Continue giving rescue breathing until—

- The child begins breathing on his or her own.
- Another trained rescuer takes over for you.
- EMS personnel arrive and take over.
- You are too exhausted to continue.

Review Questions

Check the best answer or fill in the blanks with the right word.

1. The first step in deciding whether a child needs rescue breathing is to—
   - ☐ a. Check the child's pulse.
   - ☐ b. Check for unresponsiveness.
   - ☐ c. Open the airway.

2. How do you open a child's airway?
   - ☐ a. Tilt the head gently back into the neutral-plus position and lift the chin.
   - ☐ b. Put one hand under the child's neck and tilt the head.
   - ☐ c. Push down on the chin and Adam's apple.

3. When should you give rescue breathing to a child?
   - ☐ a. When the child is breathing and has a pulse
   - ☐ b. When the child is choking
   - ☐ c. When the child is not breathing and has a pulse

4. How often should you give rescue breaths to a child?
   - ☐ a. Give 1 breath every second.
   - ☐ b. Give 1 breath every 4 seconds.
   - ☐ c. Give 1 breath every 10 seconds.

5. You should continue rescue breathing until one of four things happens. These four things are—
   - a. The child starts _____.
   - b. _____ _____ arrive and take over.
   - c. Another trained rescuer _____ _____ for you.
   - d. You are too _____ to continue.

Answers

1. **b.** The first step in deciding whether a child needs rescue breathing is to **check for unresponsiveness.**

2. **a.** To open a child's airway, **tilt the head gently back into the neutral-plus position and lift the chin.**

3. **c.** You should give rescue breathing **when the child is not breathing and has a pulse.**

4. **b.** You should give a child **1 breath every 4 seconds.**

5. You should continue rescue breathing until one of the following happens:
   a. The child starts **breathing.**
   b. **EMS personnel** arrive and take over.
   c. Another trained rescuer **takes over** for you.
   d. You are too **exhausted** to continue.

More About Rescue Breathing for a Child

Air in the Stomach

Sometimes while doing rescue breathing, you may breathe air into the child's stomach. Air in the stomach can be a serious problem because it causes the stomach to expand. Then the lungs do not have enough room to inflate when rescue breaths are given. Therefore, the child may not get enough oxygen to survive.

To avoid forcing air into the child's stomach, do the following:
- Keep the child's head in the **neutral-plus position** to keep the airway open. If you do not see the chest rise and fall with each breath, then tilt the child's head back a little farther and continue rescue breathing.
- **Give slow breaths.** Breathe at a rate of 1 to 1½ seconds for each breath.
- **Breathe only enough air to make the chest rise.** Allow the chest to fall before you give the child another breath.

Vomiting

Sometimes while you are helping an unconscious child, he or she may vomit. It is important that the stomach contents not get into the lungs. If the child vomits, quickly turn the child's head and body to either side. Wipe the material out of the child's mouth, and continue rescue breathing where you left off.

Mouth-to-Nose Breathing

There are a few situations in which you may not be able to make a good enough seal over a child's mouth to do rescue breathing. For example, the child's jaw or mouth may have been injured during an accident, or the jaw may be shut too tight to open. In such cases, mouth-to-nose breathing should be done as follows:

- Put your hand—the one nearest the child's head—on the child's forehead. Remember to tilt the child's head gently back into the neutral-plus position.
- Use your other hand to close the child's mouth by pushing on the chin *(Fig. 56).* Do not push on the throat.
- Open your mouth wide, take a deep breath, seal your mouth tightly around the child's nose, and breathe slow breaths into the nose *(Fig. 57)* at the rate of 1 to 1½ seconds for each breath. If possible, open the child's mouth between breaths by releasing the chin. This will let the air come out *(Fig. 58).*

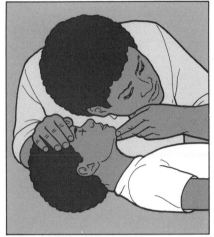

Figure 56
Close Mouth for Mouth-to-Nose Breathing

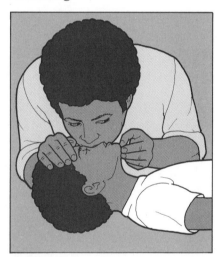

Figure 57
Mouth-to-Nose Breathing

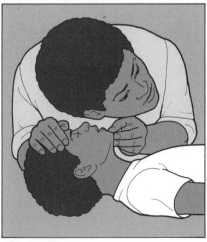

Figure 58
Check for Air Coming Out

Practice Session: Rescue Breathing for a Child

During this practice session, you and a partner will practice only on a manikin. You will practice all the steps and will give actual rescue breaths.

Before you start practicing, carefully read the skill sheet on pages 159 through 162. If you don't remember how to use the checklist, read pages 44 through 46.

Before you practice on the manikin, clean its face and the inside of its mouth. Directions for doing this are given in the section called "Some Health Precautions and Guidelines to Follow During This Course" on page 3 of this workbook. Clean the manikin's face and mouth before each person in your group practices.

Skill Sheet: Rescue Breathing for a Child

You find a child lying on the ground, not moving. You should survey the scene to see if it is safe and to get some idea of what happened. Then do a primary survey by checking the ABCs.

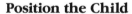

Partner Check
Instructor Check

☐ ☐ **Check for Unresponsiveness**

Tap or gently shake child's shoulder.

Rescuer shouts, "Are you OK?"

Partner/Instructor says, "Unconscious."

Rescuer repeats, "Unconscious."

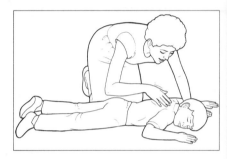

Rescuer shouts, "Help!"

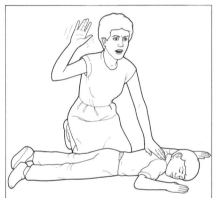

Position the Child

Roll child onto back, if necessary.

Kneel facing child, midway between child's hips and shoulders.

Straighten child's legs, if necessary, and move arm closest to you above child's head.

Lean over child and place one hand on child's shoulder and other hand on child's hip.

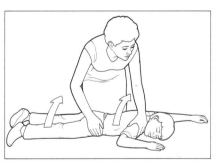

Roll child toward you as a single unit. As you roll child, move your hand from shoulder to support back of head and neck.

Place child's arm closest to you alongside child's body.

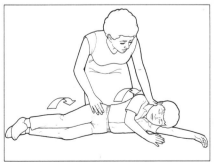

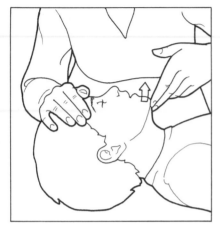

☐ ☐ **Open the Airway** (Use head-tilt/chin-lift)

Place your hand—the one nearest the child's head—on the child's forehead.

Place fingers of other hand under bony part of lower jaw at the chin.

Tilt head gently back into the neutral-plus position and lift chin. Avoid closing child's mouth completely. Avoid pushing the soft parts under the chin.

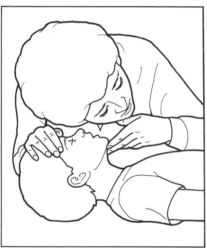

☐ ☐ **Check for Breathlessness**

Maintain open airway with head-tilt/chin-lift.

Place your ear over child's mouth and nose.

Look at chest and abdomen; listen and feel for breathing for 3 to 5 seconds.

Partner/Instructor says, "No breathing."

Rescuer repeats, "No breathing."

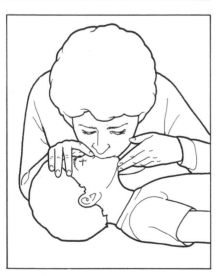

☐ ☐ **Give 2 Slow Breaths**

Maintain open airway with head-tilt/chin-lift.

Pinch nose shut.

Open your mouth wide, take a breath, and seal your lips tightly around outside of child's mouth.

Give 2 slow breaths at the rate of 1 to 1½ seconds per breath. Pause in between each breath for you to take a breath.

Look for the chest to rise and fall; listen and feel for escaping air.

Partner Check
Instructor Check

☐ ☑ **Check for Pulse**

Maintain head-tilt with one hand on forehead.

Locate Adam's apple with middle and index fingers of hand nearest child's feet.

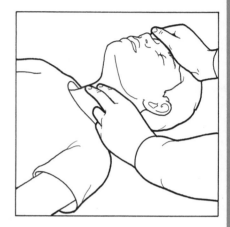

Slide fingers toward you into groove of neck on side closest to you.

Feel for carotid pulse for 5 to 10 seconds.

Partner/Instructor says, "No breathing, but there is a pulse."

Rescuer repeats, "No breathing, but there is a pulse."

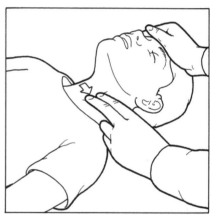

☑ ☑ **Phone the EMS System for Help**

Tell someone to call for an ambulance.

Rescuer says, "Child not breathing, has a pulse, call _____."
(Local emergency number or Operator)

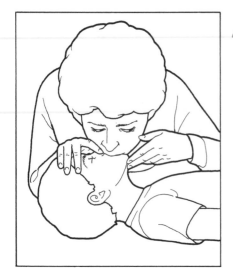

Partner Check
Instructor Check

☑ ☐ **Now Begin Rescue Breathing**

Maintain open airway with head-tilt/chin-lift.

Pinch nose shut.

Open your mouth wide, take a breath, and seal your lips tightly around outside of child's mouth.

Give 1 breath every 4 seconds at the rate of 1 to 1½ seconds per breath. Count aloud, "One one-thousand, two one-thousand, three one-thousand." Take a breath yourself and then breathe into the child.

Look for the chest to rise and fall; listen and feel for escaping air and the return of breathing.

Continue for 1 minute—about 15 breaths.

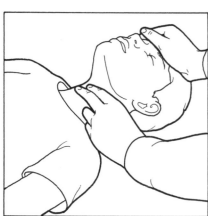

☑ ☐ **Recheck Pulse**

Maintain head-tilt with one hand on forehead.

Locate carotid pulse and feel for 5 seconds.

Partner/Instructor says, "Has a pulse."

Rescuer repeats, "Has a pulse."

Look, listen, and feel for breathing for 3 to 5 seconds.

Partner/Instructor says, "No breathing."

Rescuer repeats, "No breathing."

☑ ☐ **Continue Rescue Breathing**

Maintain open airway with head-tilt/chin-lift.

Give 1 breath every 4 seconds at the rate of 1 to 1½ seconds per breath.

Recheck pulse once every minute.

☐ ☐ **What to Do Next**

While the rescuer is rechecking pulse and breathing, the partner should read one of the following statements:
1. Child is breathing but is still unconscious.
2. Child has a pulse but is not breathing.

Based on this information, the rescuer should decide what to do next and continue giving the right care.

Final Instructor Check _____

8 *What to Do for a Child Who Is Choking*

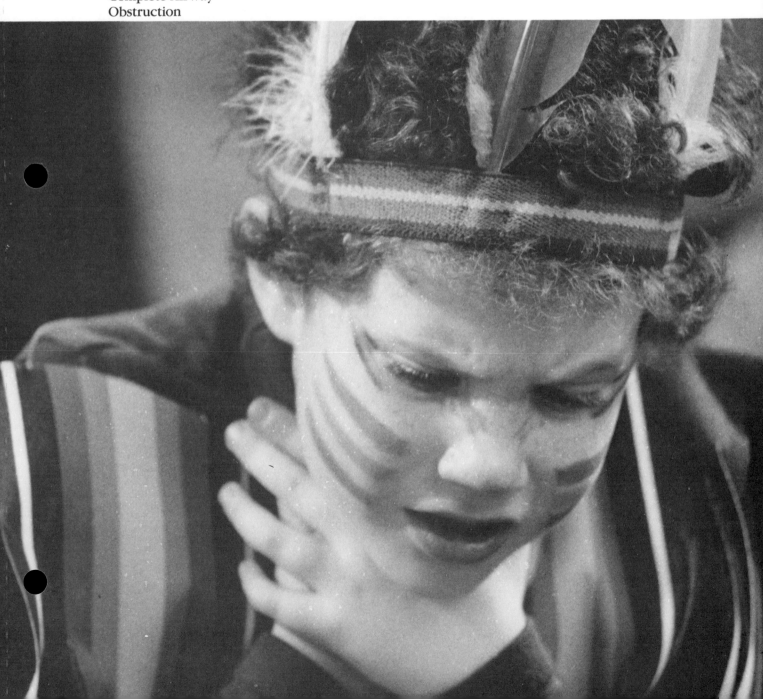

In Chapter 3, you learned first aid for an adult who is choking. In this chapter, you will learn what to do when a child is choking. When this happens, the child can quickly stop breathing, lose consciousness, and die. You will learn how to tell if a child is choking. You will learn how to tell if the child has an airway obstruction that requires first aid. You will also learn the first aid to clear an obstructed airway.

Objectives

By the time you finish reading this chapter, you should be able to do the following:

1. *Describe the signals of choking in a conscious child.*

2. *Describe the first aid for a conscious child who is choking.*

3. *Describe how you would identify an obstructed airway in an unconscious child.*

4. *Describe the first aid for an unconscious child with a complete airway obstruction.*

5. *Describe the first aid for a conscious child who becomes unconscious while choking.*

Signals of Choking

Being able to recognize when a child has an airway obstruction is the key to saving the child's life. There are two types of airway obstruction—**partial obstruction** and **complete obstruction.** It is important to be able to recognize the difference between the two.

Partial Airway Obstruction

With partial airway obstruction, the child may have either good air exchange or poor air exchange.

- When a child has **partial airway obstruction with good air exchange,** he or she can cough forcefully. **If the child is able to cough forcefully on his or her own, do not interfere with attempts to cough up the object.** You should stay with the child and encourage him or her to continue coughing. If the child keeps on coughing, call the EMS system for help.

- When a child has **partial airway obstruction with poor air exchange,** he or she may have a weak, ineffective cough, or may make a high-pitched noise like a whistling sound while breathing. An obstruction may begin with poor air exchange or it may begin with good air exchange and turn into an obstruction with poor air exchange. **Partial airway obstruction with poor air exchange should be dealt with as if it were complete airway obstruction.**

Complete Airway Obstruction

When there is complete obstruction of the airway, the child will not be able to speak, breathe, or cough. The child may appear to panic and clutch at his or her throat with one or both hands. This is the universal distress signal for choking (*Fig. 59*). You must act right away to clear the airway.

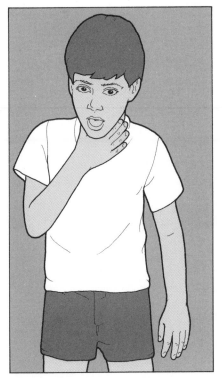

Figure 59
Universal Distress Signal for Choking

Review Questions

Check the best answer.

1. A child is choking on a piece of candy. The child is conscious and is coughing forcefully. You should—
   ☐ a. Slap the child on the back.
   ☑ b. Stay with the child and encourage him or her to continue coughing.
   ☐ c. Give the child a drink of water.

2. A conscious child is coughing weakly and is unable to speak. You should—
   ☑ a. Give first aid for complete airway obstruction.
   ☐ b. Let the child alone and watch him or her.
   ☐ c. Slap the child on the back.

Answers

1. **b.** When a conscious child is choking and is coughing forcefully, you should **stay with the child and encourage him or her to continue coughing.**

2. **a.** When a conscious child is coughing weakly and is unable to speak, you should **give first aid for complete airway obstruction.**

If don't see object don't put finger in child's mouth

First Aid for a Conscious Child With a Complete Airway Obstruction

A child should be treated as having a complete airway obstruction if—

- He or she cannot cough, speak, or breathe.
- He or she is coughing weakly or making high-pitched noises.

If you see a child who is coughing weakly and making high-pitched noises or who is unable to cough, speak, or breathe, you should survey the scene as you approach the child.

1. Begin a primary survey by asking, "Are you choking?"

2. If you are alone, shout for help.

3. Tell the child that you are trained in first aid and can help. Have someone phone the EMS system for help.

4. Do abdominal thrusts (sometimes called the Heimlich maneuver) as follows:
   - Stand or kneel behind the child. The child should be standing or sitting. Wrap your arms around his or her waist. Make a fist with one hand. Place the thumb side of your fist against the middle of the child's abdomen, just above the navel and well below the lower tip of the breastbone (*Figs. 60, 61, and 62*).

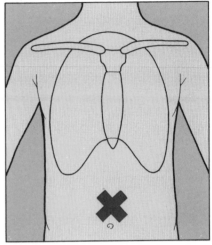

Figure 60
Location for Abdominal Thrusts

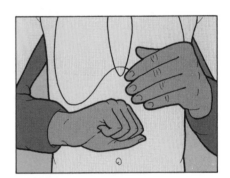

Figure 61
Location for Abdominal Thrusts

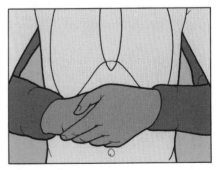

Figure 62
Hand Placement for Abdominal Thrusts

- Grasp your fist with your other hand. Keeping your elbows out from the child, press your fist into the child's abdomen with a quick upward thrust (*Fig. 63*). Be sure that your fist is directly on the midline of the child's abdomen when you press. Do not direct the thrusts to the right or to the left. Think of each thrust as a separate and distinct attempt to dislodge the object.
- Repeat the thrusts until the obstruction is cleared or until the child becomes unconscious.

Later in this chapter, you will learn how to help a choking child who becomes unconscious.

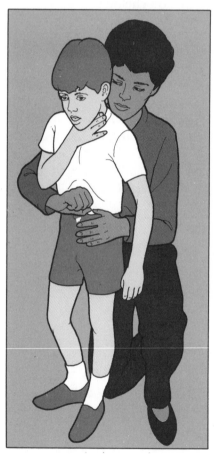
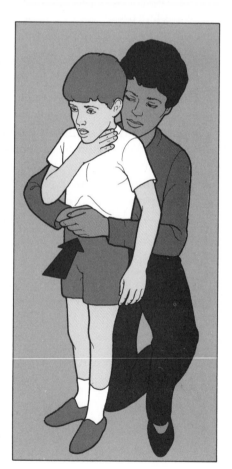

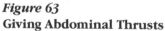
Figure 63
Giving Abdominal Thrusts

When to Stop

Immediately stop giving thrusts if the object is coughed up or the child starts to breathe or cough. Watch the child, and make sure that the child is breathing freely again. Even after the child coughs up the object, he or she may have breathing problems that will need a doctor's attention. You should also realize that abdominal thrusts may cause internal injuries. For these reasons, you should call the EMS system if you have not already done so. **The child should be taken to the hospital emergency department even if he or she seems to be breathing well.**

Review Questions

Check the best answer(s).

3. You recognize that a conscious child is choking. When should you give abdominal thrusts? (Check all that apply.)
   - ☒ a. When the child is coughing weakly or making high-pitched noises
   - ☐ b. When the child is coughing forcefully
   - ☒ c. When the child is unable to cough, speak, or breathe

4. When you give abdominal thrusts to a conscious child, what position should the child be in?
   - ☐ a. Lying on his or her back
   - ☒ b. Sitting or standing with his or her back to you
   - ☐ c. Standing and facing you

5. When you give abdominal thrusts to a conscious child, what part of your fist should you place against the child?
   - ☐ a. The palm side
   - ☒ b. The thumb side
   - ☐ c. The knuckles

6. When you give abdominal thrusts to a conscious child, where should you place your fist?
   - ☐ a. At the lower tip of the breastbone
   - ☒ b. Just above the navel and well below the lower tip of the breastbone
   - ☐ c. On the navel

7. Abdominal thrusts should be given to a conscious child—
   - ☒ a. With a quick upward thrust.
   - ☐ b. With a downward thrust.
   - ☐ c. With a slow inward pressure.

Answers

3. a. Abdominal thrusts should be given **when the child is coughing weakly or making high-pitched noises.**
  c. Abdominal thrusts should be given **when the child is unable to cough, speak, or breathe.**

4. b. When you give abdominal thrusts to a conscious child, the child should be **sitting or standing with his or her back to you.**

5. b. When you give abdominal thrusts to a conscious child, you should place **the thumb side** of your fist against the child.

6. b. When you give abdominal thrusts to a conscious child, you should place your fist **just above the navel and well below the lower tip of the breastbone.**

7. a. Abdominal thrusts should be given to a conscious child **with a quick upward thrust.**

First Aid for an Unconscious Child With a Complete Airway Obstruction

First aid for any unconscious child begins with a primary survey. While checking the ABCs, you may find that the child has an obstructed airway. The procedure for identifying a complete airway obstruction in an unconscious child is given below. You should start by surveying the scene and then do a primary survey.

1. Check for unresponsiveness.
2. Shout for help.
3. Position the child on his or her back.
4. Open the airway.
5. Look, listen, and feel for breathing.
6. If the child is not breathing, give 2 slow breaths.
7. If you are unable to breathe air into the child, retilt the head and give 2 more breaths. You may not have tilted the child's head into the correct position the first time.

If you still cannot breathe air into the child, tell someone to phone the EMS system for help and do the following:

8. Give 6 to 10 abdominal thrusts (as explained on page 172).
9. Do a foreign-body check (as explained on pages 172 and 173).
10. Open the airway and give 2 slow breaths.

Repeat steps 8, 9, and 10 until the obstruction is cleared or EMS personnel arrive and take over.

Abdominal Thrusts

To give abdominal thrusts to an unconscious child—

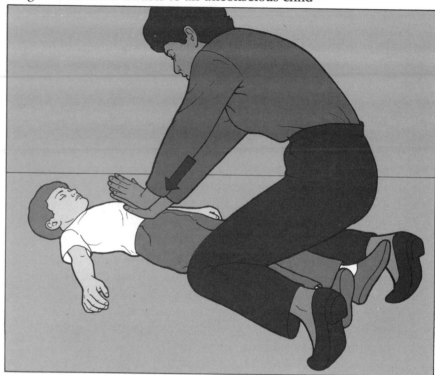

Figure 64
Abdominal Thrusts for Unconscious Child

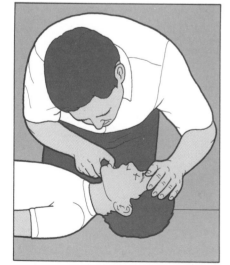

Figure 65
Location for Abdominal Thrusts

- Kneel at the child's feet. If the child is large, straddle the child, as you would an adult victim **(Fig. 64)**.
- Place the heel of one hand against the middle of the child's abdomen, just above the navel and well below the lower tip of the breastbone **(Fig. 65)**. Put your other hand on top of your first hand with the fingers of both hands pointed toward the child's head. Do not allow your fingers to press on the child's ribs.
- Press into the abdomen with a quick upward thrust. Give 6 to 10 thrusts. Be sure that your hands are directly on the midline of the abdomen when you press. Do not direct the thrusts to the right or to the left. Each thrust should be a separate attempt to dislodge the object. After you have given 6 to 10 abdominal thrusts, do a foreign-body check to find out if the object has been dislodged. A description of the foreign-body check follows.

Foreign-Body Check

To do a foreign-body check—
- Kneel beside the child's head.
- Open the child's mouth using the hand that is nearest the child's feet. Put your thumb into the mouth and grasp both the tongue and the lower jaw between your thumb and fingers. Lift the jaw upward **(Fig. 66)**. This lifts the tongue away from the back of the throat and away from any object that may be lodged there.

Figure 66
Foreign-Body Check

172

- Look for the object. If you can see an object, try to remove it with the finger sweep *(Figs. 67, 68).*

Note: To do the finger sweep, slide the little finger of your other hand into the child's mouth. Slide your finger down along the inside of the cheek to the base of the child's tongue. Be careful not to push the object deeper into the airway. Use a hooking action to sweep the object out of the throat.

Remember: Do the finger sweep only if you can see the object in the child's throat.

Give 2 Slow Breaths

After you do the foreign-body check, give 2 slow breaths, as follows:
- Open the airway with the head-tilt/chin-lift.
- Give 2 slow breaths.

Continue these three steps:
1. Give 6 to 10 abdominal thrusts.
2. Do a foreign-body check.
3. Open the airway and give 2 slow breaths.

If your first attempts to clear the airway are unsuccessful, do not stop. The longer the child goes without oxygen, the more the muscles of the throat will relax, making it more likely that you will be able to remove the foreign body.

If you succeed in clearing the airway and are able to breathe air into the child, give 2 slow breaths, as you did for rescue breathing. Then check the child's pulse. If there is no pulse, begin CPR. You will learn how to do CPR for a child in Chapter 9. If there is a pulse and the child is not breathing on his or her own, continue rescue breathing.

If the child starts breathing on his or her own, monitor breathing and pulse until EMS personnel arrive and take over. This means you should maintain an open airway; look, listen, and feel for breathing; and keep checking the pulse. Also, cover the child, and keep him or her warm and as quiet as possible.

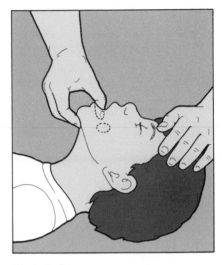

Figure 67
Grasp Tongue and Lower Jaw

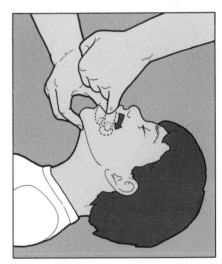

Figure 68
Finger Sweep for a Child

Put the Steps Together

Here is the whole procedure for an unconscious child who may have a complete airway obstruction:

1. Check for unresponsiveness.
2. Shout for help.
3. Position the child on his or her back.
4. Open the airway.
5. Look, listen, and feel for breathing.
6. Give 2 slow breaths.
7. Retilt the head if you are unable to breathe air into the child.
8. Give 2 slow breaths.

If you are still unable to breathe air into the child's lungs, have someone phone the EMS system for help and—

9. Give 6 to 10 abdominal thrusts.
10. Do a foreign-body check.
11. Open the child's airway and give 2 slow breaths.

Repeat steps 9, 10, and 11 until the obstruction is cleared or EMS personnel arrive and take over. If you succeed in removing the object, open the airway and give 2 slow breaths. Then check for a pulse. If there is no pulse, begin CPR. If there is a pulse, check for breathing. If the child is not breathing on his or her own, continue rescue breathing.

Review Questions

Check the best answer(s).

8. A child is unconscious and is not breathing. If you cannot breathe air into the child's lungs when you give the first 2 breaths, what should you do next?
   - ☒ a. Retilt the child's head.
   - ☐ b. Look in the mouth for an object blocking the airway.
   - ☐ c. Give 6 to 10 abdominal thrusts.

9. When you are giving abdominal thrusts to an unconscious child, what position should the child be in?
   - ☒ a. Lying on his or her back
   - ☐ b. Lying on his or her side
   - ☐ c. Lying on his or her stomach

10. How should you position yourself when you are giving abdominal thrusts to an unconscious child? (Check all that apply.)
    - ☐ a. Kneel by the child's chest.
    - ☐ b. Kneel by the child's head.
    - ☒ c. Kneel beside the child's feet.
    - ☒ d. Straddle the child's legs if the child is large.

11. To give abdominal thrusts to an unconscious child, you should place the heel of one hand—
    - ☐ a. Over the edge of the rib cage.
    - ☒ b. In the middle of the child's abdomen just above the navel and well below the lower tip of the breastbone.
    - ☐ c. Directly over the navel.

12. How should you give abdominal thrusts to an unconscious child?
    - ☐ a. With a downward thrust
    - ☐ b. With a slow inward pressure
    - ☒ c. With a quick upward thrust

13. How many abdominal thrusts should you give to an unconscious child before doing a foreign-body check?
    - ☐ a. 1 to 3
    - ☒ b. 6 to 10
    - ☐ c. 15 to 20

14. After removing an object from a child's mouth, you give the child 2 breaths and see the chest rise and fall. What should you do next?
    - ☐ a. Open the airway.
    - ☒ b. Check the pulse.
    - ☐ c. Phone the EMS system for help.

Answers

8. a. You should **retilt the child's head** if you cannot breathe air into the lungs of an unconscious child who is not breathing.

9. a. When you are giving abdominal thrusts to an unconscious child, the child should be **lying on his or her back.**

10. c. When you are giving abdominal thrusts to an unconscious child, you should **kneel beside the child's feet.**

 d. When you are giving abdominal thrusts to an unconscious child, you should **straddle the child's legs if the child is large.**

11. b. You should place the heel of one hand **in the middle of the child's abdomen just above the navel and well below the lower tip of the breastbone** to give abdominal thrusts to an unconscious child.

12. c. You should give abdominal thrusts to an unconscious child **with a quick upward thrust.**

13. b. You should give **6 to 10** abdominal thrusts to an unconscious child before doing a foreign-body check.

14. b. When you see the child's chest rise and fall, you should **check the pulse.**

First Aid for Choking When a Conscious Child Becomes Unconscious

Sometimes a child with a complete airway obstruction may lose consciousness and fall. If this happens, you should shout for help and slowly lower the child to the floor while supporting the child from behind. Support the child's head as you lower the child to the floor.

Once the child is on the floor, tell someone to phone the EMS system for help if it hasn't already been done. Then kneel beside the child and do the following:

1. Do a foreign-body check.
2. Open the airway and give 2 slow breaths.
3. Give 6 to 10 abdominal thrusts if you are unable to breathe into the child's lungs.

Repeat these three steps until the obstruction is cleared or EMS personnel arrive and take over.

Practice Session: First Aid for a Child Who Is Choking (Complete Airway Obstruction)

The first aid for a child who is choking is the same as the first aid for an adult who is choking. Since you have already practiced these skills on a partner or a manikin, you are not required to practice them again. However, you should read the two skill sheets in this chapter: First Aid for a Conscious Child With a Complete Airway Obstruction and First Aid for an Unconscious Child With a Complete Airway Obstruction. These skill sheets may be used if your instructor asks you to practice.

Skill Sheet: First Aid for a Conscious Child With a Complete Airway Obstruction

Remember: **While practicing abdominal thrusts on a partner or a child, pretend to give thrusts. Never give abdominal thrusts to someone who is not choking.**

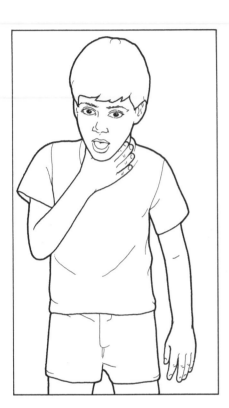

Determine If Child Is Choking

Rescuer asks, "Are you choking?"

Partner/Instructor says, "Child cannot cough, speak, or breathe."

Rescuer shouts, "Help!"

Phone the EMS System for Help

Tell someone to call for an ambulance.

Rescuer says, "Child choking, call _____."
(Local emergency number or Operator)

Perform Abdominal Thrusts

Stand or kneel behind child.

Wrap arms around child's waist.

Make a fist with one hand and place thumb side of fist against middle of child's abdomen just above navel and well below lower tip of breastbone.

Grasp your fist with your other hand.

Keeping elbows out away from child, press fist into child's abdomen with a quick upward thrust.

Each thrust should be a separate and distinct attempt to dislodge the object.

Repeat thrusts until obstruction is cleared or child becomes unconscious.

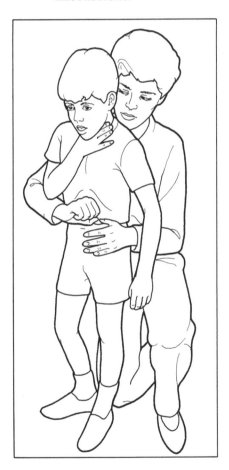 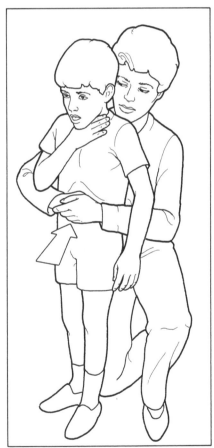

Skill Sheet: First Aid for an Unconscious Child With a Complete Airway Obstruction

You find a child lying on the ground, not moving. You should survey the scene to see if it is safe and to get some idea of what happened. Then do a primary survey by checking the ABCs.

Remember: **Do not do finger sweeps on a manikin. Do not touch the manikin's lips or inside the mouth with your fingers.**

Check for Unresponsiveness
Tap or gently shake child's shoulder.

Rescuer shouts, "Are you OK?"

Partner/Instructor says, "Unconscious."

Rescuer repeats, "Unconscious."

Rescuer shouts, "Help!"

Position the Child

Roll child onto back, if necessary.

Kneel facing child, midway between child's hips and shoulders.

Straighten child's legs, if necessary, and move child's arm closest to you above child's head.

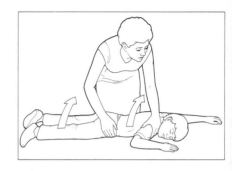

Lean over child and place one hand on child's shoulder and other hand on child's hip.

Roll child toward you as a single unit. As you roll child, move your hand from child's shoulder to support back of head and neck.

Place child's arm closest to you alongside child's body.

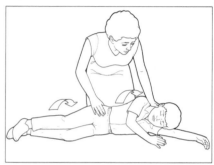

Open the Airway (Use head-tilt/chin-lift)

Place your hand—the one nearest the child's head—on child's forehead.

Place fingers of other hand under bony part of lower jaw near chin.

Tilt head gently back into the neutral-plus position and lift chin. Avoid closing child's mouth completely. Avoid pushing on the soft parts under the chin.

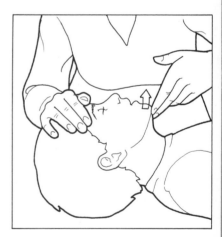

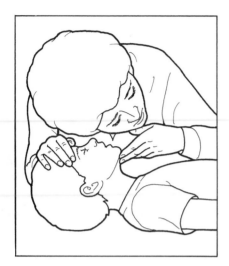

Check for Breathlessness

Maintain open airway with head-tilt/chin-lift.

Place your ear over child's mouth and nose.

Look at chest and abdomen; listen and feel for breathing for 3 to 5 seconds.

Partner/Instructor says, "No breathing."

Rescuer repeats, "No breathing."

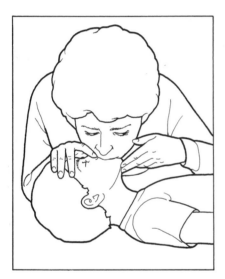

Give 2 Slow Breaths

Maintain open airway with head-tilt/chin-lift.

Pinch nose shut.

Open your mouth wide, take a breath, and seal your lips tightly around outside of child's mouth.

Give 2 slow breaths at the rate of 1 to 1½ seconds per breath. Pause in between each breath for you to take a breath.

Partner/Instructor says, "Unable to breathe air into child."

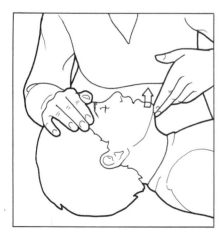

Retilt Child's Head and Give 2 Slow Breaths

Retilt child's head and lift chin. Avoid closing child's mouth completely. Avoid pushing on the soft parts under the chin.

Pinch nose shut.

Open your mouth wide, take a breath, and seal your lips tightly around outside of child's mouth.

Give 2 slow breaths at the rate of 1 to 1½ seconds per breath. Pause in between each breath for you to take a breath.

Partner/Instructor says, "Still unable to breathe air into child."

Rescuer says, "Airway obstructed."

Phone the EMS System for Help

Tell someone to call for an ambulance.

Rescuer says, "Child's airway obstructed, call _____."

(Local emergency number or Operator)

Perform 6 to 10 Abdominal Thrusts

Leave child faceup on his or her back.

Kneel at child's feet or straddle child's legs.

Locate child's navel.

Place heel of one hand on middle of child's abdomen just above navel and well below the lower tip of the breastbone.

Place other hand directly on top of first hand. (Fingers of both hands should be pointing toward child's head.)

Press into child's abdomen 6 to 10 times with quick upward thrusts.

Each thrust should be a separate and distinct attempt to dislodge the object.

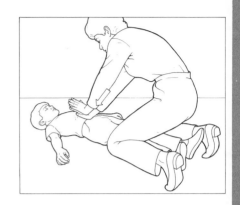

Foreign-Body Check

Move from child's feet and kneel beside child's head.

With child's face up, open the mouth and grasp both tongue and lower jaw between thumb and fingers of hand nearest child's legs. Lift jaw.

Look inside mouth for object. If object is visible, attempt to remove it with a finger sweep.

Partner/Instructor says, "No object seen."

Rescuer repeats, "No object seen."

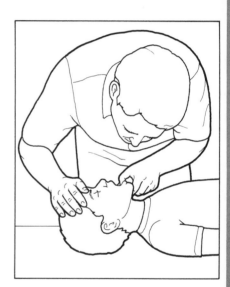

Give 2 Slow Breaths

Maintain open airway with head-tilt/chin-lift.

Pinch nose shut.

Open your mouth wide, take a breath, and seal your lips tightly around outside of child's mouth.

Give 2 slow breaths at the rate of 1 to 1½ seconds per breath. Pause in between each breath for you to take a breath.

Partner/Instructor says, "Airway still obstructed."

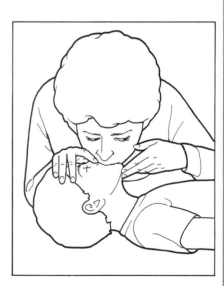

Repeat Sequence

Perform 6 to 10 abdominal thrusts.

Do foreign-body check.

Give 2 slow breaths.

What to Do Next

While the rescuer is repeating the sequence of abdominal thrusts, foreign-body check, and rescue breaths, the partner should read one of the following statements:

1. Rescuer can breathe into child's lungs after doing foreign-body check.
2. After foreign-body check, object is removed with finger sweep.
3. Object is expelled during abdominal thrusts.

Based on this information, the rescuer should decide what to do next and continue giving the right care.

9 What to Do When a Child's Heart Stops (CPR)

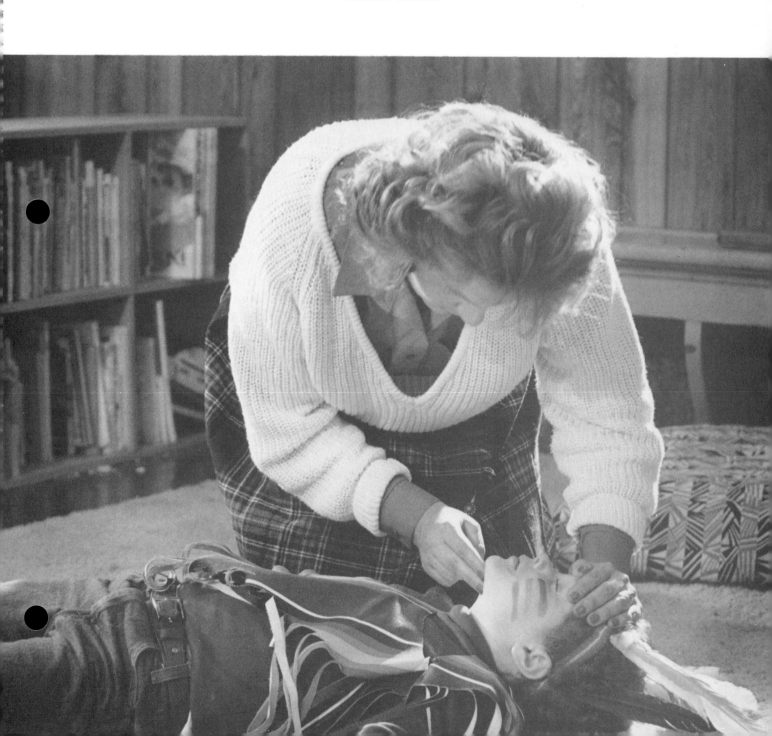

In Chapter 5, you learned how to give CPR to an adult. In this chapter, you will learn how to give CPR to a child age one through eight. When a child's heart stops, his or her survival depends on how quickly CPR is started and how quickly he or she receives advanced emergency medical care.

In this chapter, you will learn what to do for a child whose heart has stopped beating. You will learn how to keep oxygen-carrying blood moving through the child's body.

Objectives

By the time you finish reading this chapter, you should be able to do the following:

1. *Describe the early signals of a cardiac emergency.*
2. *Recognize when a child needs CPR.*
3. *Explain why it is important to check the child's carotid pulse before you start CPR.*
4. *Describe how to give CPR to a child.*
5. *Describe when you should check for the return of the child's pulse after you start CPR.*
6. *List four conditions when a rescuer may stop CPR.*

Cardiac Emergencies in Children

Children's hearts are usually healthy. Unlike adults, children do not often initially suffer a cardiac emergency. In most cases, the child first suffers a respiratory emergency. Then a cardiac emergency develops.

The most common cause of cardiac emergencies in children is injury resulting from motor vehicle accidents. Other common causes include injuries resulting from near-drowning, smoke inhalation, burns, poisoning, airway obstruction, firearms, and falls. Rarely, a cardiac emergency can result from a medical condition or illness such as severe croup, severe asthma, or respiratory infections such as epiglottitis.

Most cardiac emergencies in children are preventable. One way to prevent cardiac emergencies is to prevent children from being injured. In Chapter 6, you read about how you can reduce the risk of injury. Second, it is important to make sure children receive proper medical care. A third preventive measure is learning to recognize the early signals of a respiratory emergency since a cardiac emergency often results from a respiratory emergency. These signals may include any of the following:

- Agitation
- Drowsiness
- Change in skin color (to pale, blue, or gray)
- Increased difficulty in breathing
- Increased heart and breathing rates

In this chapter, you will learn how to give first aid to a child who has suffered a cardiac emergency. When a cardiac emergency does happen, you should immediately begin first aid as described in this chapter.

How to Give CPR to a Child

To find out if a child needs CPR, begin with a primary survey to check the ABCs. You should—
1. Check for unresponsiveness.
2. Shout for help.
3. Position the child on his or her back.
4. Open the airway.
5. Look, listen, and feel for breathing.
6. If the child is not breathing, give 2 slow breaths.
7. Check the carotid pulse.
8. Have someone phone the EMS system for help.

If the child has no pulse, begin CPR. **It is important to check the child's carotid pulse for 5 to 10 seconds before you start CPR because it is dangerous to do chest compressions if the child's heart is beating.**

To give CPR, kneel beside the child, lean over the chest, and find the correct position to give chest compressions. Give chest compressions and rescue breaths. These two steps keep oxygen-carrying blood flowing through the blood vessels.

Locating the Compression Position

For chest compressions to work, the child must be lying flat on his or her back on a firm, flat surface. The child's head must be on the same level as the heart.

To give effective compressions, your hands and body must be in the correct position. Do the following:

- Kneel beside the child's chest with your knees against the child's side.
- Use your hand—the one nearest the child's head—to keep the child's head in the neutral-plus position.
- Use your other hand—the one nearest the child's legs—to find the lower edge of the rib cage on the child's side closest to you. Slide your middle finger up the edge of the rib cage to the notch where the ribs meet the breastbone in the center of the lower part of the chest (*Figs. 69, 70*). Put your middle finger in this notch, with the index finger beside it (*Fig. 71*). The two fingers should be resting on the lower end of the breastbone.

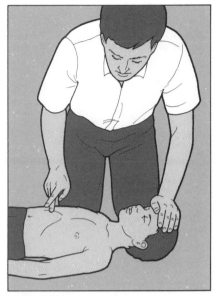

Figure 69
Slide Finger up Edge of Rib Cage

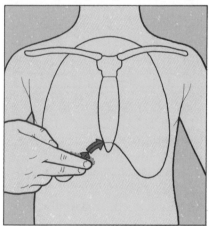

Figure 70
Find Correct Position

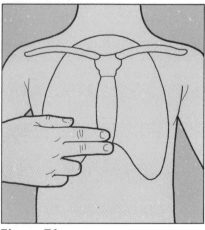

Figure 71
Position Fingers on Breastbone

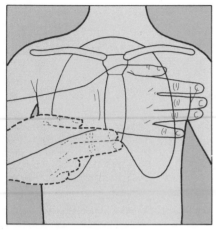

Figure 72
**Place Heel of Hand on
Breastbone**

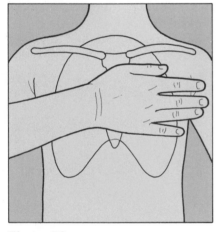

Figure 73
Lift Fingers off Breastbone

• Pay attention to where you put your index finger.
Lift your fingers off the breastbone, and put the heel of the same hand on the breastbone immediately above where you had your index finger (*Fig. 72*). Keep your fingers off the child's chest. Only the heel of your hand should rest on the breastbone (*Fig. 73*). Use this method to find the correct hand position before you begin compressions.

Having your hands in the correct position will lessen the chance of fracturing the ribs on either side of the child's breastbone. It also keeps you from pushing the tip of the breastbone into the delicate organs beneath it.

Review Questions

Check the best answer.

1. The first step in finding the proper hand position to give chest compressions to a child is to—
   - ☒ a. Slide your middle finger up the edge of the rib cage to the notch where the ribs meet the breastbone.
   - ☐ b. Find the top of the breastbone.
   - ☐ c. Find the navel.

2. When your hand is in the correct compression position, your fingers should be—
   - ☐ a. Resting on the child's chest.
   - ☒ b. Held off the child's chest.
   - ☐ c. Curling into your palm.

Answers

1. **a.** The first step in finding the proper hand position to give chest compressions to a child is to **slide your middle finger up the edge of the rib cage to the notch where the ribs meet the breastbone.**

2. **b.** When your hand is in the correct compression position, your fingers should be **held off the child's chest.**

Body Position of Rescuer

The position of your body is very important when you are giving compressions. You should be kneeling beside the child. After you have placed your hand in the correct position to give compressions, move your body until your shoulder is directly over your hand. In this position, when you push down, you will be pushing straight down onto the breastbone. Your other hand should be on the child's forehead, keeping the child's head in the neutral-plus position (*Fig. 74*).

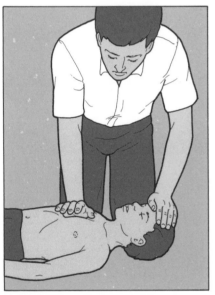

Figure 74
Correct Position of Rescuer

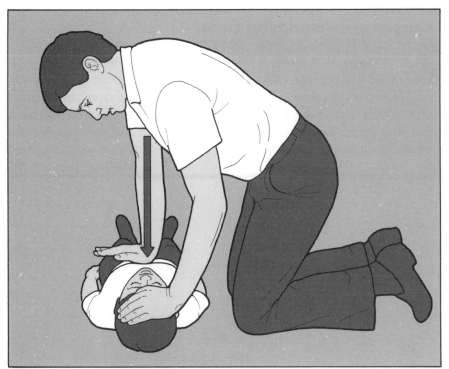

Figure 75
Giving Chest Compressions

Compression Technique

This is how you give chest compressions to a child:

1. When you compress, use only the hand that is on the child's breastbone. You will **not** use both hands to give chest compressions to a child as you practiced for an adult. Push straight down. If you rock back and forth and don't push straight down, your compressions will not be effective (*Fig. 75*).

2. Each compression should push the breastbone down from 1 to 1½ inches (2.5 to 3.8 centimeters) (*Fig. 76*). The down-and-up movement should be smooth, not jerky. Keep a steady down-and-up rhythm, and do not pause between compressions. Half the time should be spent pushing down, and half the time should be spent coming up. When you are coming up, release pressure on the chest completely, but don't lift your hand off the child's chest. Keep your hand in the compression position.

3. Give compressions at the rate of 80 to 100 compressions per minute.

4. Take note of the position your hand is in so you can remember it. When you take your hand off the child's chest, put it back in the same position before you start compressions again. You do not have to find the position each time by sliding your finger up the rib cage.

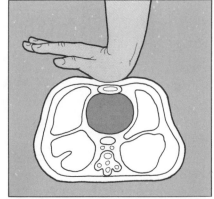

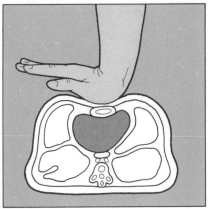

Figure 76
Compress Chest 1 to 1½ Inches

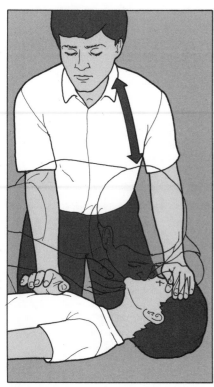

Figure 77
5 Compressions, Then 1 Breath

Compression/Breathing Cycles

When you give CPR, do cycles of 5 compressions and 1 breath (*Fig.* 77). In each cycle, give 5 compressions with one hand. Keep your other hand on the child's forehead, tilting the head so that it is in the neutral-plus position. Then remove your hand from the chest, lift the chin, and give 1 breath. Always stop compressions to lift the chin and give 1 breath. After you give the breath, put your hand back on the chest in the correct position.

Put the Steps Together

Here are the steps you should follow when you give CPR to a child:

1. Check for unresponsiveness.
2. Shout for help.
3. Make sure that the child is on his or her back on a firm, flat surface.
4. Open the airway.
5. Look, listen, and feel for breathing (3 to 5 seconds).
6. If the child is not breathing, give 2 slow breaths.
7. Check the child's carotid pulse for heartbeat (5 to 10 seconds).
8. Tell someone to phone the EMS system for help.
9. If there is no pulse, locate the correct hand position and position yourself to give chest compressions.
10. Give 5 compressions without stopping at the rate of 80 to 100 compressions per minute, counting out loud, "One and two and three and four and five and." Push down as you say the number and come up as you say the "and." Remember to keep your other hand on the child's forehead keeping the head in the neutral-plus position.
11. Next, lift the chin, and give 1 slow breath. The breath should take about 1 to 1½ seconds.
12. Keep repeating—5 compressions, 1 breath, 5 compressions, 1 breath, and so on. The complete cycle of 5 compressions and 1 breath should take from 4 to 6 seconds.
13. Recheck pulse. After you do 10 cycles (or about 1 minute) of continuous CPR, check to see if the child has a pulse. Do this after you give the breath at the end of the 10th cycle of 5 compressions and 1 breath. Check the carotid pulse at the neck for 5 seconds. If there is no pulse, give 1 breath and continue CPR. Repeat the pulse check every few minutes.

    If you do find a pulse, then check for breathing for 3 to 5 seconds. If the child is breathing, keep the airway open and monitor breathing and pulse closely. This means that you should look, listen, and feel for breathing. Check the pulse once every minute. Cover the child, and keep the child warm and as quiet as possible. If the child is not breathing, give rescue breathing and keep checking the pulse.
14. Continue CPR until one of these things happens:
    - The heart starts beating again.
    - A second rescuer trained in CPR takes over for you.
    - EMS personnel arrive and take over.
    - You are too exhausted to continue.

More About CPR for a Child

If No One Comes When You Shout for Help

When you determine that a child is unconscious, always shout for help immediately. Your shout may attract someone who can phone the EMS system for help. But what if no one responds to your shouts for help? You should do CPR for 1 minute. During this minute you should continue to shout for help. You should also use this minute to plan how to make the call yourself.

If no one has responded to your shouts for help by the end of 1 minute of CPR, you should get to a phone as quickly as you can and call the EMS system. If possible, you should bring the phone to the area where the child is or carry the child with you to the phone. Then begin CPR again.

If a Second Trained Rescuer Is at the Scene

If another rescuer trained in CPR is at the scene, this person should do two things: first, phone the EMS system for help if this has not been done; second, take over CPR when the first rescuer is tired. Here are the steps for entry of the second rescuer:

- The second person should identify himself or herself as a CPR-trained rescuer who is willing to help.
- If the EMS system has been called and if the first rescuer is tired and asks for help, then—

  1. The first rescuer should stop CPR after the next breath.

  2. The second rescuer should kneel next to the child opposite the first rescuer, tilt the head into the neutral-plus position, and feel for the carotid pulse for 5 seconds.

  3. If there is no pulse, the second rescuer should give 1 breath and continue CPR.

  4. The first rescuer should then check the adequacy of the second rescuer's breaths and chest compressions. This is done by watching the child's chest rise and fall during rescue breathing, and by feeling the carotid pulse for an artificial pulse during chest compressions. This artificial pulse will tell you that blood is moving through the body.

Review Questions

Check the best answer or fill in the blanks with the right word.

3. While you are giving compressions with one hand, where should your other hand be?
   - ☐ a. Under the child's shoulders
   - ☐ b. Under the child's head and neck
   - ☑ c. On the child's forehead, keeping the head in the neutral-plus position

4. How far should you compress the chest of a child?
   - ☐ a. ½ to 1 inch (1.3 to 2.5 centimeters)
   - ☑ b. 1 to 1½ inches (2.5 to 3.8 centimeters)
   - ☐ c. 1½ to 2 inches (3.8 to 5 centimeters)

5. At what rate should you compress the chest when you give CPR to a child?
   - ☐ a. 50 to 60 times per minute
   - ☐ b. 60 to 80 times per minute
   - ☑ c. 80 to 100 times per minute

6. After giving a breath, you should replace your hand on the child's chest by—
   - ☐ a. Putting your hand back on the breastbone in the correct position.
   - ☐ b. Sliding your finger up the lower edge of the rib cage to the notch at the lower end of the breastbone.

7. When you give CPR to a child, what is the ratio of compressions to breaths?
   - ☑ a. 5 compressions, then 1 breath
   - ☐ b. 10 compressions, then 2 breaths
   - ☐ c. 12 compressions, then 5 breaths

8. After starting CPR on a child, how often should you check for the return of pulse?
   - ☐ a. After 5 minutes and every 5 to 6 minutes thereafter
   - ☐ b. After 2 minutes and every 4 to 5 minutes thereafter
   - ☑ c. After 1 minute and every few minutes thereafter

9. What are the four conditions when you may stop CPR?
   a. When the heart starts _beating_ again.
   b. When a second rescuer trained in _CPR_ takes over for you.
   c. When _EMS_ personnel arrive and take over.
   d. When you are too _tired_ to continue.

Answers

3. c. While you are giving compressions with one hand, your other hand should be **on the child's forehead, keeping the head in the neutral-plus position.**

4. b. You should compress the chest of a child **1 to 1½ inches (2.5 to 3.8 centimeters).**

5. c. When you give CPR to a child, you should compress the chest at the rate of **80 to 100 times per minute.**

6. a. You should replace your hand on the child's chest by **putting your hand back on the breastbone in the correct position.**

7. a. When you give CPR to a child, the ratio is **5 compressions, then 1 breath.**

8. c. After starting CPR on a child, check for the return of pulse **after 1 minute and every few minutes thereafter.**

9. You may stop CPR—
   a. When the heart starts **beating** again.
   b. When a second rescuer trained in **CPR** takes over for you.
   c. When **EMS** personnel arrive and take over.
   d. When you are too **exhausted** to continue.

Practice Session: CPR for a Child

During this practice session, you and a partner will practice only on a manikin.

Before you start practicing, carefully read the skill sheet on pages 197 through 206. If you don't remember how to use the checklist, read pages 44 through 46.

Before you practice on the manikin, clean its face and the inside of its mouth. Directions for doing this are given in the section called "Some Health Precautions and Guidelines to Follow During This Course" on page 3 of this workbook. Clean the manikin's face and mouth before each person in your group practices.

Skill Sheet: CPR for a Child

You find a child lying on the ground, not moving. You should survey the scene to see if it is safe and to get some idea of what happened. Then do a primary survey by checking the ABCs.

Partner Check
Instructor Check

☐☐ **Check for Unresponsiveness**
Tap or gently shake child's shoulder.

Rescuer shouts, "Are you OK?"

Partner/Instructor says, "Unconscious."

Rescuer repeats, "Unconscious."

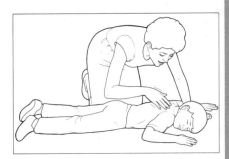

Rescuer shouts, "Help!"

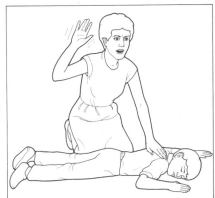

Position the Child
Roll child onto back, if necessary.

Kneel facing child, midway between child's hips and shoulders.

Straighten child's legs, if necessary, and move child's arm closest to you above child's head.

Lean over child and place one hand on child's shoulder and other hand on child's hip.

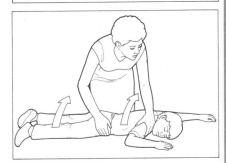

Roll child toward you as a single unit. As you roll child, move your hand from child's shoulder to support back of head and neck.

Place child's arm closest to you alongside child's body.

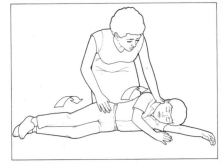

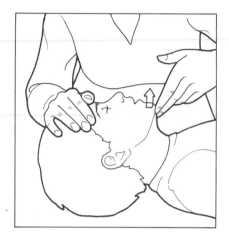

Open the Airway (Use head-tilt/chin-lift)

Place your hand—the one nearest child's head—on child's forehead.

Place fingers of other hand under bony part of lower jaw at the chin.

Tilt head gently back into the neutral-plus position and lift chin. Avoid closing child's mouth completely. Avoid pushing on the soft parts under the chin.

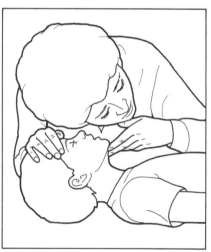

Check for Breathlessness

Maintain open airway with head-tilt/chin-lift.

Place your ear over child's mouth and nose.

Look at chest and abdomen; listen and feel for breathing for 3 to 5 seconds.

Partner/Instructor says, "No breathing."

Rescuer repeats, "No breathing."

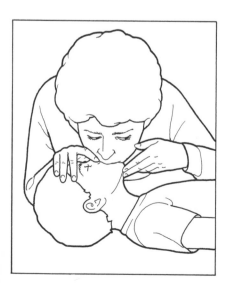

Give 2 Slow Breaths

Maintain open airway with head-tilt/chin-lift.

Pinch nose shut.

Open your mouth wide, take a breath, and seal your lips tightly around outside of child's mouth.

Give 2 slow breaths at the rate of 1 to 1½ seconds per breath. Pause in between each breath for you to take a breath.

Look for the chest to rise and fall; listen and feel for escaping air.

Partner Check
Instructor Check

☑ ☑ **Check for Pulse**

Maintain head-tilt with one hand on forehead.

Locate Adam's apple with middle and index fingers of your hand nearest child's feet.

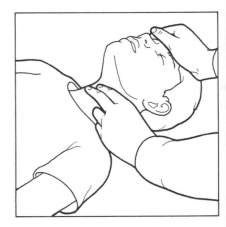

Slide fingers toward you into groove of neck on side closest to you.

Feel for carotid pulse for 5 to 10 seconds.

Partner/Instructor says, "No breathing and no pulse."

Rescuer repeats, "No breathing and no pulse."

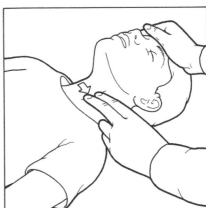

☑ ☑ **Phone the EMS System for Help**

Tell someone to call for an ambulance.

Rescuer says, "Child not breathing, has no pulse, call _____."

(Local emergency number or Operator)

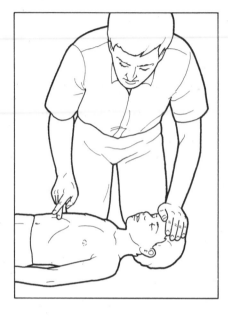

Partner Check   Instructor Check

☐ ☐ **Locate Compression Position**

Kneel facing child's chest.

Maintain head-tilt with hand on forehead.

With middle finger of hand nearest child's legs, locate lower edge of child's rib cage on side closest to you.

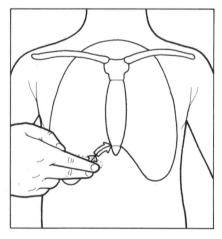

Slide middle finger up edge of rib cage to notch at lower end of breastbone.

Place middle finger in notch and index finger next to it on lower end of breastbone.

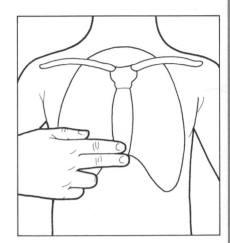

Look at where your index finger is placed on child's breastbone.

Lift fingers off breastbone.

Place heel of same hand on breastbone immediately above where index finger was placed.

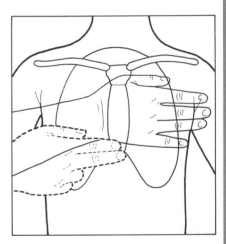

Keep fingers off child's chest.

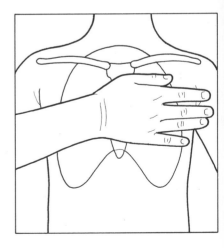

one hand

5 compressions

1 breath

After 10 cycles ch. pulse

Partner Check

Instructor Check

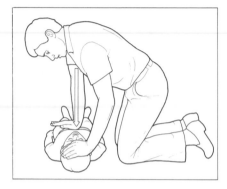

Position shoulder over hand.

Give 5 Compressions

Compress breastbone 1 to 1½ inches (2.5 to 3.8 centimeters) at a rate of 80 to 100 compressions per minute. (5 compressions should take 3 to 4 seconds.)

Count aloud, "One and two and three and four and five and." (Push down as you say the number and come up as you say "and.")

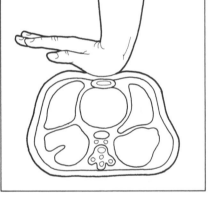

Compress down and up smoothly, keeping hand contact with chest at all times.

Maintain head-tilt with hand on forehead.

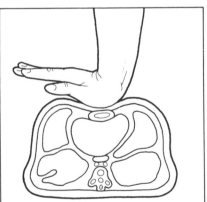

☐ ☐ **Give 1 Slow Breath**

Maintain head-tilt with hand on forehead.

Place fingers of other hand under bony part of lower jaw at the chin. Lift chin.

Pinch nose shut.

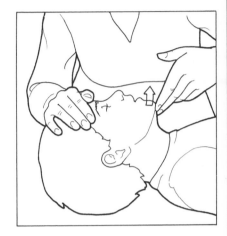

Open your mouth wide, take a breath, and seal your lips tightly around outside of child's mouth.

Give 1 slow breath (lasting 1 to 1½ seconds).

Look for chest to rise and fall; listen and feel for escaping air.

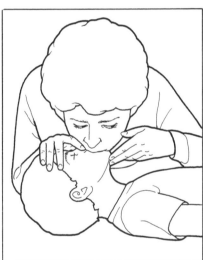

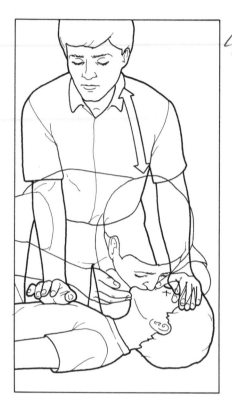

Partner Check

Instructor Check

☐ ☐ **Do Compression/Breathing Cycles**

Maintain head-tilt with hand on forehead.

Return hand doing chin-lift directly to compression position.

Do 10 cycles of 5 compressions and 1 breath.

Partner Check
Instructor Check

☐ ☐ **Recheck Pulse**
Maintain head-tilt with one hand on forehead.

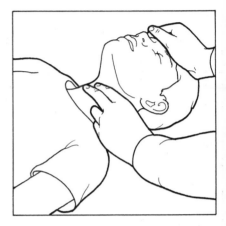

Feel for carotid pulse for 5 seconds.

Partner/Instructor says, "No pulse."

Rescuer repeats, "No pulse."

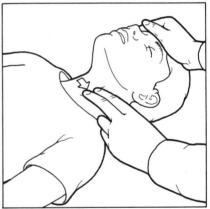

Partner Check
Instructor Check

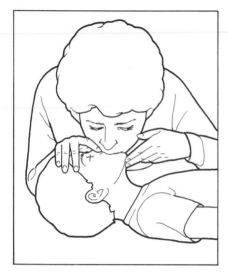

☑ ☑ **Give 1 Slow Breath**

Maintain head-tilt with hand on forehead.

Pinch nose shut.

Place fingers of other hand under bony part of lower jaw at the chin. Lift chin.

Open your mouth wide, take a breath, and seal your lips tightly around outside of child's mouth.

Give 1 slow breath (lasting 1 to 1½ seconds).

Look for the chest to rise and fall; listen and feel for escaping air.

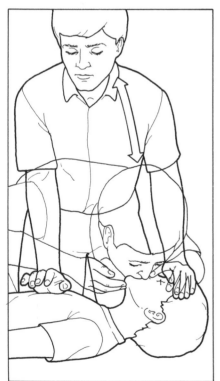

☑ ☐ **Continue Compression/Breathing Cycles**

Return hand to compression position.

Continue cycles of 5 compressions and 1 breath.

Recheck pulse every few minutes.

☐ ☐ **What to Do Next**

When the rescuer stops to check pulse, the partner should read one of the following statements:

1. Child has a pulse.
2. Child does not have a pulse.

Based on this information, the rescuer should decide what to do next and continue giving the right care.

Final Instructor Check _____

10

What to Do When an Infant's Breathing Stops (Rescue Breathing)

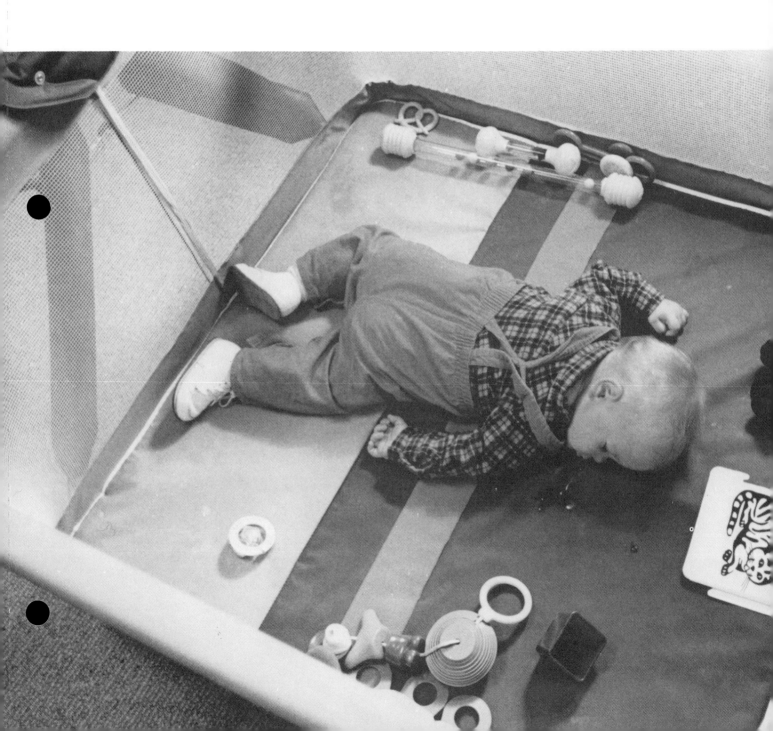

In Chapter 7, you learned rescue breathing for a child. To give rescue breathing to an infant, you need to learn a different technique. In this chapter, you will learn rescue breathing for an infant newborn to age one.

Objectives

By the time you finish reading this chapter, you should be able to do the following:

1. Describe the early signals of a respiratory emergency.
2. Describe when an infant needs rescue breathing.
3. Describe how to position an infant for rescue breathing.
4. Describe how to give rescue breathing to an infant.

Respiratory Emergencies in Infants

Rescue breathing is given to an infant whose breathing has stopped but whose heart is still beating. Injuries resulting from motor vehicle accidents, poisoning, airway obstruction, suffocation, smoke inhalation, burns, and near-drowning can cause a respiratory emergency. A respiratory emergency can also be the result of a medical condition or illness such as severe croup, or respiratory infections such as epiglottitis, or severe bronchiolitis.

It is important to recognize the early signals of a respiratory emergency. These signals may include any of the following:

- Agitation
- Drowsiness
- Changes in skin color (to pale, blue, or gray)
- Increased difficulty in breathing
- Increased heart and breathing rates

If an infant displays any of these signs, you should begin first aid as described in this chapter. By recognizing a potential respiratory emergency and/or dealing with one when it occurs, you may prevent a cardiac emergency from happening.

How to Give Rescue Breathing to an Infant

If you find an infant lying very still, and you suspect that something might be wrong, you should quickly survey the scene and do a primary survey.

1. **Check for Unresponsiveness**

   The first thing you should do is check to see if the infant is conscious. Tap or gently shake the infant's shoulder to see if he or she responds (*Fig. 78*).

2. **Shout for Help**

   If the infant does not move or make a noise, shout for help. You do this to get the attention of people you can ask to phone the EMS system for help after you complete a primary survey (*Fig. 79*).

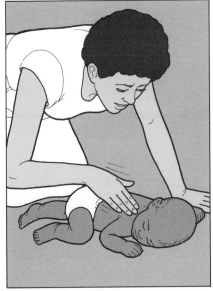

Figure 78
Check for Unresponsiveness

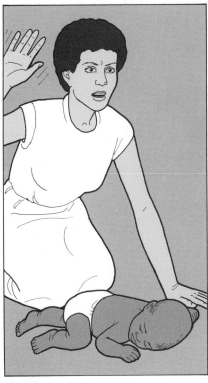

Figure 79
Shout for Help

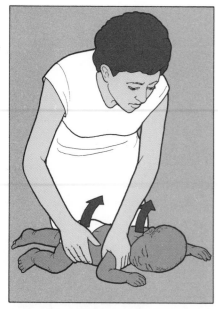

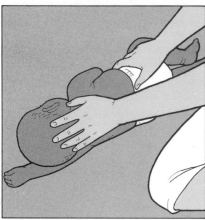

Figure 80
Position the Infant

3. Position the Infant

Move the infant onto his or her back. To do this, roll the infant as a unit (*Fig. 80*). This will help to avoid twisting the body and making any injuries worse. To position the infant—

- Stand or kneel facing the infant.
- Straighten the infant's legs, if necessary.
- Move the infant's arm closest to you so that it is stretched out above the infant's head.
- Lean over the infant and place one hand on the infant's shoulder and the other on the infant's hip.
- Roll the infant toward you as a single unit by pulling slowly and evenly.
- As you roll the infant onto his or her back, move your hand from the shoulder to support the back of the head and neck.
- Put the infant's arm closest to you alongside the infant's body.

It is important to position the infant on his or her back as quickly as possible. It should take no more than 10 seconds to do this.

Note: Some infants who require rescue breathing or CPR may have received a serious injury to the head, neck, or back. Moving these infants or opening the airway as described below may result in further injury. Additional methods for handling these infants are discussed in the American Red Cross CPR: Basic Life Support for the Professional Rescuer course.

4. "A"—Open the Airway

Immediately open the infant's airway using the head-tilt/chin-lift *(Fig. 81)*. This is the most important action you can take to help the infant survive. To open the airway—

- Stand or kneel beside the infant's head.
- Put your hand—the one nearest the infant's head—on the infant's forehead.
- Put one finger (not the thumb) of your other hand under the bony part of the infant's lower jaw at the chin.
- Tilt the infant's head back into the neutral position by applying pressure on the forehead and lifting the chin. The neutral position is shown in *Figure 82.* Don't close the infant's mouth completely. Don't push in on the soft parts under the chin.

5. "B"—Check for Breathlessness (Look, listen, and feel for breathing.)

With the infant's head in the neutral position and the chin lifted, check to see if the infant is breathing *(Fig. 83)*. Tilting the head into the neutral position and lifting the chin opens the airway and may in itself restore breathing. To check the infant's breathing—

- Place your ear just over the infant's mouth and nose and look at the infant's chest and abdomen.
- Look, listen, and feel. **Look** for the chest and abdomen to rise and fall, **listen** for breathing, and **feel** for air coming out of the infant's nose and mouth against your ear and cheek. Do this for 3 to 5 seconds.

If the infant is breathing, you will see the chest and abdomen move, and you will hear and feel air escaping at your ear and cheek. Movement of the chest and abdomen does not always mean that the infant is breathing. He or she may be making unsuccessful attempts to breathe. Be sure to look, listen, and feel for breathing.

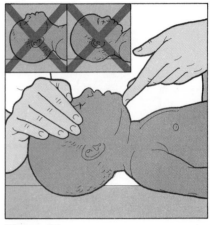

Figure 81
Tilt Head Into Neutral Position and Lift Chin

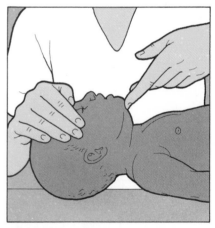

Figure 82
Head-Tilt/Chin-Lift

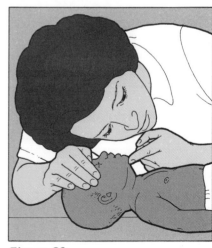

Figure 83
Check for Breathlessness

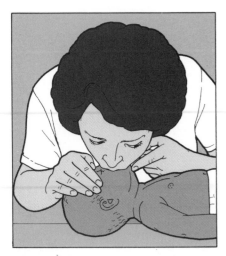

Figure 84
Mouth-to-Mouth-and-Nose Breathing

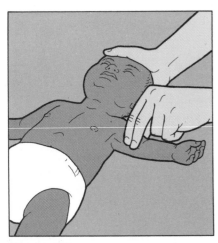

Figure 85
Locate Brachial Pulse

6. **Give 2 Slow Breaths**

   If the infant is not breathing, you must get air into the lungs at once *(Fig. 84).* To give breaths—
   - Keep the airway open with the head-tilt/chin-lift. Open your mouth wide, take a breath, and seal your lips tightly around the infant's mouth and nose.
   - Give 2 slow breaths at the rate of 1 to 1½ seconds per breath. Remove your mouth between breaths just long enough for you to take a breath. Watch for the chest to rise while you breathe into the infant. Watch for the chest to fall after each breath. Listen and feel for air escaping as the infant's chest falls.

   If air does not go into the infant's lungs, retilt the head and give 2 more breaths. If air still does not go into the infant's lungs, the airway may be blocked by food or some other material. Chapter 11 describes how to help an infant with an airway obstruction.

   Because the infant's airway is smaller than an adult's, it may be difficult to breathe air into the lungs. Be careful not to breathe too hard. If you blow too fast and too forcefully into the infant's airway, you can cause air to go into the stomach. On the other hand, if you blow too softly, you will not fill the infant's lungs with air. You should breathe slowly and watch for the chest to rise. When the chest rises, stop breathing into the infant.

7. **"C"—Check Circulation by Checking for a Pulse in the Upper Arm**

   Check to see if the infant's heart is beating by feeling for a pulse in the upper arm closest to you. This pulse is called the **brachial pulse** *(Fig. 85).* It is located on the inside of the upper arm between the elbow and the shoulder. To check for a brachial pulse—
   - Keep one hand on the infant's forehead to keep the head in the neutral position.
   - Use your other hand to find the pulse. Place your thumb on the outside of the infant's arm closest to you. Press gently with your index and middle fingers on the inside of the arm between the elbow and shoulder.
   - Feel for the brachial pulse with your fingers for 5 to 10 seconds.

8. **Phone the EMS System**

   After you have checked the pulse, you will have enough information about the infant's condition to give to the bystanders you are sending to phone the EMS system. Tell them whether the infant is conscious, breathing, and has a pulse. Tell them to give this information to the EMS dispatcher.

9. Begin Rescue Breathing

If you feel a pulse and the infant is not breathing, then begin rescue breathing. (If you do not feel a pulse, the infant's heart has stopped, and you must start CPR, which you will learn in Chapter 12.) To give rescue breathing—

- Keep the infant's airway open using the head-tilt/chin-lift.
- Open your mouth wide, take a breath, and seal your lips tightly around the infant's mouth and nose. Give 1 breath every 3 seconds. Each breath should last for 1 to 1½ seconds. A good way to time the breaths is to count, "One one-thousand, two one-thousand." Take a breath yourself and then breathe into the infant. Watch for the chest to rise as you breathe into the infant.
- Between breaths, remove your mouth from the infant. Look for the chest to fall as you listen and feel at the infant's mouth and nose for escaping air. Listen to hear if the infant starts breathing again.

10. Recheck Pulse

After 1 minute of rescue breathing (about 20 breaths), you should check the infant's pulse. To check the pulse—

- Keep the infant's head in the neutral position with one hand on the forehead.
- With the other hand, feel for the brachial pulse for 5 seconds.

If the infant has a pulse, then check for breathing for 3 to 5 seconds.

If the infant is breathing, keep the airway open and monitor breathing and pulse closely. This means that you should look, listen, and feel for breathing. Keep checking the pulse once every minute. Cover the infant, and keep the infant warm and as quiet as possible.

If the infant is not breathing, continue rescue breathing and keep checking the pulse once every minute. Continue giving rescue breathing until—

- The infant begins breathing on his or her own.
- Another trained rescuer takes over for you.
- EMS personnel arrive and take over.
- You are too exhausted to continue.

Review Questions

Check the best answer or fill in the blanks with the correct word.

1. You find an infant lying very still on the floor. You survey the scene and decide it is safe. What should you do when you reach the infant?
   - ☒ a. Check for unresponsiveness.
   - ☐ b. Check the infant's pulse.
   - ☐ c. Open the airway.
   - ☐ d. Immediately begin rescue breathing.

2. When should you give rescue breathing to an infant?
   - ☐ a. When the infant is breathing and has a pulse
   - ☐ b. When the infant's heart has stopped beating
   - ☒ c. When the infant is not breathing and has a pulse

3. Where should you place your fingers when doing the chin-lift on an infant?
   - ☐ a. Under the back of the infant's neck
   - ☐ b. In the groove between the windpipe and the muscle at the side of the neck
   - ☒ c. Under the bony part of the lower jaw at the chin

4. Where should you check for an infant's brachial pulse?
   - ☐ a. In the groove between the windpipe and the muscle at the side of the neck
   - ☐ b. On the thumbside of the wrist
   - ☑ c. On the inside of the upper arm between the elbow and the shoulder

5. How often should you give rescue breaths to an infant?
   - ☐ a. Give 1 breath every second.
   - ☑ b. Give 1 breath every 3 seconds.
   - ☐ c. Give 1 breath every 10 seconds.

6. You should continue rescue breathing until one of four things happens. These four things are—
   a. The infant starts _breath_.
   b. _EMS_ _arrive_ arrive and take over.
   c. Another trained rescuer _takes_ _over_ for you.
   d. You are too _exhausted_ to continue.

Answers

1. **a.** If you find an infant lying unusually still, the first thing you should do is **check for unresponsiveness.**

2. **c.** You should give rescue breathing to an infant **when the infant is not breathing and has a pulse.**

3. **c.** When doing the chin-lift on an infant, you should place your fingers **under the bony part of the lower jaw at the chin.**

4. **c.** You should check for an infant's brachial pulse **on the inside of the upper arm between the elbow and the shoulder.**

5. **b.** For an infant, **give 1 breath every 3 seconds.**

6. You should continue rescue breathing until one of the following happens:
   a. The infant starts **breathing.**
   b. **EMS personnel** arrive and take over.
   c. Another trained rescuer **takes over** for you.
   d. You are too **exhausted** to continue.

More About Rescue Breathing for an Infant

Air in the Stomach

Sometimes while doing rescue breathing, you may breathe air into the infant's stomach. Air in the stomach can be a serious problem because it causes the stomach to expand. Then the lungs do not have enough room to inflate when rescue breaths are given. Therefore, the infant may not get enough oxygen to survive.

To avoid forcing air into the infant's stomach, do the following:

- Keep the infant's head in the **neutral position** to keep the airway open. If you feel that the air is not going in easily, then tilt the infant's head back a little farther and continue rescue breathing.
- **Give slow breaths**. Breathe at a rate of 1 to 1½ seconds for each breath.
- **Breathe only enough air to make the chest rise.** Allow the chest to fall before you give the infant another breath.

Vomiting

Sometimes while you are helping an unconscious infant, he or she may vomit. It is important that the stomach contents not get into the lungs. If the infant vomits, quickly turn the infant's head and body to either side. Wipe the material out of the infant's mouth, and continue rescue breathing where you left off.

Practice Session: Rescue Breathing for an Infant

During this practice session, you and a partner will practice only on a manikin. You will practice all the steps and will give actual rescue breaths.

Before you start practicing, carefully read the skill sheet on pages 218 through 222. If you don't remember how to use the checklist, read pages 44 through 46.

Before you practice on the manikin, clean its face and the inside of its mouth. Directions for doing this are given in the section called "Some Health Precautions and Guidelines to Follow During This Course" on page 3 of this workbook. Clean the manikin's face and mouth before each person in your group practices.

Skill Sheet: Rescue Breathing for an Infant

You find an infant lying unusually still, and you suspect that something may be wrong. You should survey the scene to see if it is safe and to get some idea of what happened. Then do a primary survey by checking the ABCs.

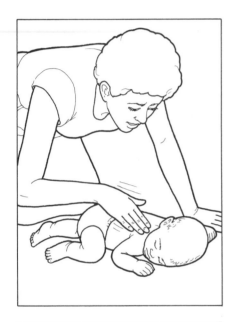

☐ ☑ **Check for Unresponsiveness**
Tap or gently shake infant's shoulder.

Partner/Instructor says, "Unconscious."

Rescuer repeats, "Unconscious."

Rescuer shouts, "Help!"

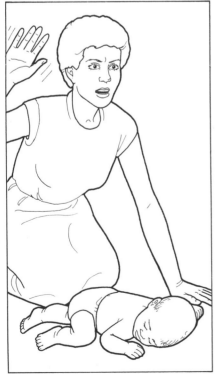

Position the Infant

Roll infant onto back, if necessary.

Stand or kneel facing infant.

Straighten infant's legs, if necessary, and move infant's arm closest to you above infant's head.

Lean over infant and place one hand on infant's shoulder and other hand on infant's hip.

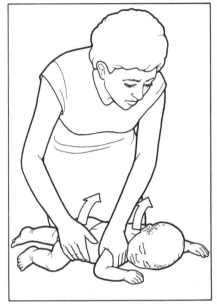

Roll infant toward you as a single unit. As you roll infant, move your hand from infant's shoulder to support back of head and neck.

Place infant's arm closest to you alongside infant's body.

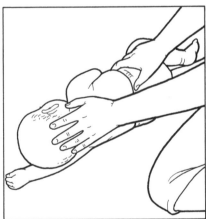

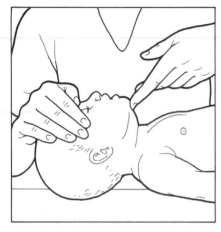

Partner Check

Instructor Check

☐ ☑ **Open the Airway** (Use head-tilt/chin-lift)

Place your hand—the one nearest the infant's head—on infant's forehead.

Place finger of other hand under bony part of lower jaw at the chin.

Tilt head gently back into the neutral position and lift chin. Avoid closing infant's mouth completely. Avoid pushing on the soft parts under the chin.

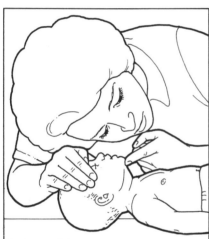

☐ ☑ **Check for Breathlessness**

Maintain open airway with head-tilt/chin-lift.

Place your ear over infant's mouth and nose.

Look at chest and abdomen; listen and feel for breathing for 3 to 5 seconds.

Partner/Instructor says, "No breathing."

Rescuer repeats, "No breathing."

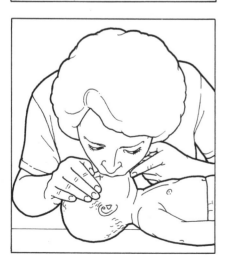

☑ **Give 2 Slow Breaths**

Maintain open airway with head-tilt/chin-lift.

Open your mouth wide, take a breath, and seal your lips tightly around infant's mouth and nose.

Give 2 slow breaths at the rate of 1 to 1½ seconds per breath. Pause in between each breath for you to take a breath.

Look for the chest to rise and fall; listen and feel for escaping air.

Partner Check
Instructor Check

☐ ☑ **Check for Pulse**

Maintain head-tilt with one hand on forehead.

Place thumb of other hand on outside of infant's upper arm closest to you. Your thumb should be halfway between the shoulder and elbow. Press gently with your index and middle fingers on inside of arm.

Feel for brachial pulse for 5 to 10 seconds.

Partner/Instructor says, "No breathing, but there is a pulse."

Rescuer repeats, "No breathing, but there is a pulse."

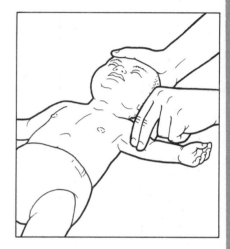

☐ ☑ **Phone the EMS System for Help**

Tell someone to call for an ambulance.

Rescuer says, "Infant not breathing, has a pulse, call _____."
(*Local emergency number or Operator*)

☐ ☑ **Now Begin Rescue Breathing**

Maintain open airway with head-tilt/chin-lift.

Open your mouth wide, take a breath, and seal your lips tightly around infant's mouth and nose.

Give 1 breath every 3 seconds at the rate of 1 to 1½ seconds per breath. Count aloud, "One one-thousand, two one-thousand." Take a breath yourself and then breathe into the infant.

Look for the chest to rise and fall; listen and feel for escaping air and the return of breathing.

Continue for 1 minute—about 20 breaths.

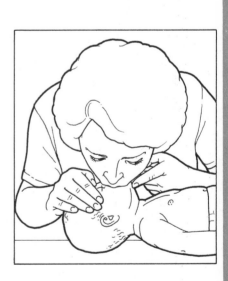

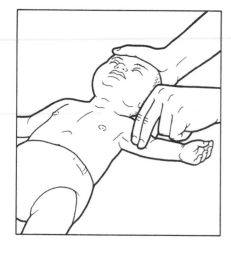

Partner Check
Instructor Check

Continue for 1 min

☐ ☑ **Recheck Pulse**

Maintain head-tilt with one hand on forehead.

Locate brachial pulse and feel for 5 seconds.

Partner/Instructor says, "Has a pulse."

Rescuer repeats, "Has a pulse."

Look, listen, and feel for breathing for 3 to 5 seconds.

Partner/Instructor says, "No breathing."

Rescuer repeats, "No breathing."

☐ ☑ **Continue Rescue Breathing**

Maintain open airway with head-tilt/chin-lift.

Give 1 breath every 3 seconds at the rate of 1 to 1½ seconds per breath.

Recheck pulse once every minute.

☐ ☐ **What to Do Next**

While the rescuer is rechecking pulse and breathing, the partner should read one of the following statements:

1. Infant is breathing but is still unconscious.

2. Infant has a pulse but is not breathing.

Based on this information, the rescuer should decide what to do next and continue giving the right care.

Final Instructor Check _____

11 *What to Do for an Infant Who Is Choking*

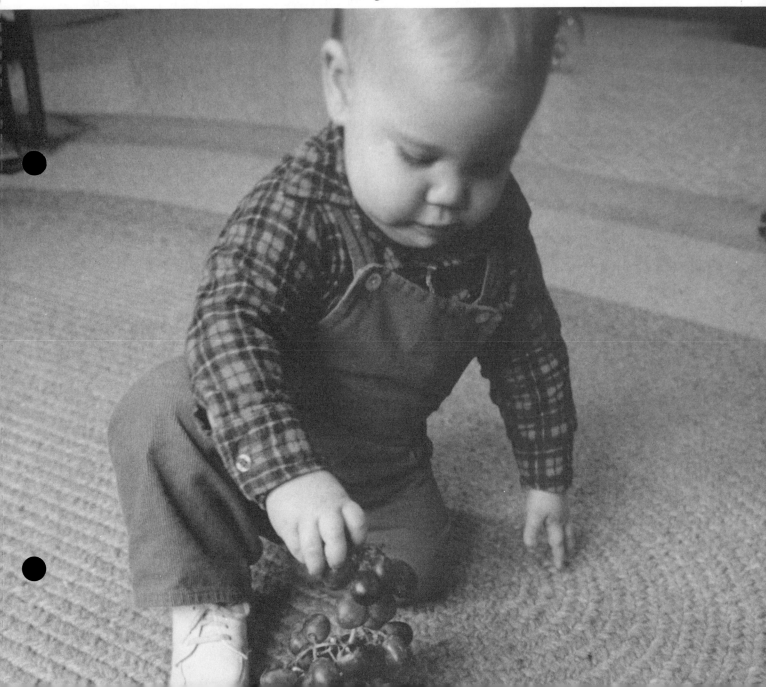

In Chapter 8, you learned first aid for a child who is choking. In this chapter, you will learn what to do when an infant is choking. When this happens, the infant can quickly stop breathing, lose consciousness, and die. In this chapter, you will learn how to tell if an infant has an airway obstruction that requires first aid. You will also learn the first aid to clear an obstructed airway.

Objectives

By the time you finish reading this chapter, you should be able to do the following:

1. *Describe the signals of choking in a conscious infant.*
2. *Describe the first aid for a conscious infant who is choking.*
3. *Describe how you would identify an obstructed airway in an unconscious infant.*
4. *Describe the first aid for an unconscious infant with a complete airway obstruction.*
5. *Describe the first aid for a conscious infant who becomes unconscious while choking.*

Causes and Signals of Choking

As you read in Chapter 6, one way infants explore their world is by putting objects in their mouth. This is one reason why choking is a major cause of death in infants. Infants also are likely to choke because they develop their eating skills gradually. First they suck from a bottle or breast; then they are fed soft foods. Finally they grow teeth and learn to feed themselves a variety of foods. But foods that an adult can eat easily, such as nuts or popcorn, can cause an infant to choke.

When a piece of food or an object such as a coin lodges in an infant's airway, the infant can quickly stop breathing, become unconscious, and die. For this reason, it is important to recognize the signals of choking so you can give immediate first aid. There are two types of airway obstruction—**partial obstruction** and **complete obstruction.** It is important to be able to recognize the difference between the two.

Partial Airway Obstruction
With partial airway obstruction, the infant may have either good air exchange or poor air exchange.
- When an infant has **partial airway obstruction with good air exchange,** he or she can cough forcefully. **If the infant is able to cough forcefully on his or her own, do not interfere with attempts to cough up the object.** Watch the infant carefully. If the infant keeps on coughing, call the EMS system for help.
- When an infant has **partial airway obstruction with poor air exchange,** he or she may have a weak, ineffective cough, or may make a high-pitched noise like a whistling sound while breathing. An obstruction may begin with poor air exchange or it may begin with good air exchange and turn into an obstruction with poor air exchange. **Partial airway obstruction with poor air exchange should be dealt with as if it were complete airway obstruction.**

Complete Airway Obstruction
When there is complete obstruction of the airway, the infant will not be able to breathe, cough, or cry. You must act right away to clear the airway.

Review Questions

Check the best answer.

1. An infant is choking on some food. She is conscious and is coughing forcefully on her own. You should—
   - ☐ a. Do abdominal thrusts.
   - ☑ b. Watch the infant carefully.
   - ☐ c. Pat the infant gently on the back.

2. A conscious infant is coughing weakly and making a whistling sound when he breathes. You should—
   - ☑ a. Give first aid for complete airway obstruction.
   - ☐ b. Watch the infant carefully.
   - ☐ c. Do abdominal thrusts.

Answers

1. **b.** If a choking infant is conscious and is coughing forcefully, you should **watch the infant carefully.**

2. **a.** You should **give first aid for complete airway obstruction** if a conscious infant is coughing weakly and making a whistling sound when he breathes.

First Aid for a Conscious Infant With a Complete Airway Obstruction

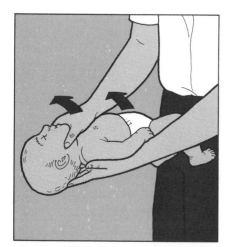

Figure 86
Hold Infant's Jaw

An infant should be treated as having a complete airway obstruction if—
- He or she cannot cough, breathe, or cry.
- He or she is coughing weakly or making high-pitched noises.

   If you suspect that an infant is choking, you should survey the scene as you approach the infant.

1. Begin a primary survey. Determine if the infant can cough, breathe, or cry.
2. If you are alone, shout for help.
3. Have someone phone the EMS system for help.
4. Give 4 back blows as follows:
   - Hold the infant's jaw between your thumb and fingers *(Fig. 86)*.
   - Slide your other hand behind the infant's shoulder blade closest to you so that your fingers support the back of the infant's head and neck.
   - Turn the infant over so that he or she is facedown on your forearm *(Fig. 87)*.
   - Support infant's head and neck with your hand by firmly holding the jaw between your thumb and fingers.

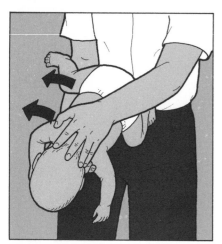

Figure 87
Turn Infant Over

- Lower your arm onto your thigh. The infant's head should be lower than his or her chest.
- Give 4 back blows forcefully between the infant's shoulder blades with the heel of your hand *(Fig. 88)*.

5. Then give 4 chest thrusts as follows:
   - Place your free hand and forearm along infant's head and back so that the infant is sandwiched between your two hands and forearms.
   - Support the back of the infant's head and neck with your fingers *(Fig. 89)*.

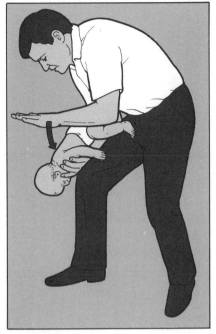

Figure 88
Give 4 Back Blows

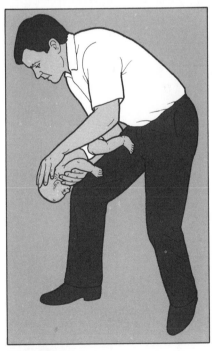

Figure 89
Support Back of Infant's Head and Neck

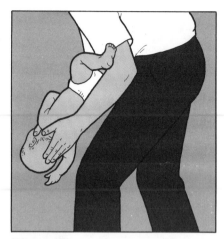

Figure 90
Turn Infant Onto Back

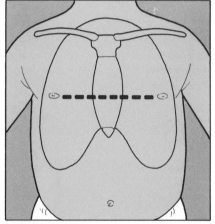

Figure 91
Imaginary Line Between Nipples

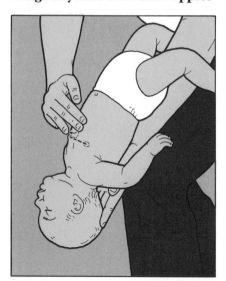

Figure 92
Locate Position for Chest Thrusts

- Support the infant's neck, jaw, and chest from the front with one hand while you support the infant's back with your other hand and forearm.
- Turn the infant onto his or her back *(Fig. 90)*.
- Lower your arm that is supporting the infant's back onto your thigh. The infant's head should be lower than his or her chest. (If the infant is large or your hands are too small to support the infant, put the infant on your lap with his or her head lower than the chest.)
- Use your hand that is on the infant's chest to locate the correct place to give chest thrusts. Imagine a line running across the infant's chest between the nipples *(Fig. 91)*. Place the pad of your ring finger on the breastbone just under this imaginary line *(Fig. 92)*. Then place the pads of two fingers next to the ring finger just under the nipple line. Raise the ring finger. If you feel the notch at the end of the infant's breastbone, move your fingers up a little bit. The pads of your fingers should lie in the same direction as the infant's breastbone.
- Use the pads of two fingers to compress the breastbone *(Fig. 93)*. Compress the breastbone ½ to 1 inch (1.3 to 2.5 centimeters), and then let the breastbone return to its normal position. Keep your fingers in contact with the infant's breastbone. Compress 4 times.

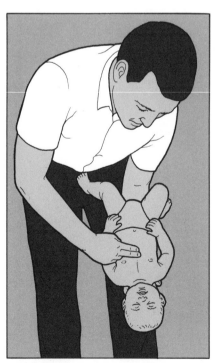

Figure 93
Position for Giving Chest Thrusts

- Keep giving the infant back blows and chest thrusts until the object is coughed up or the infant loses consciousness.

Later in this chapter, you will learn how to help a choking infant who becomes unconscious.

When to Stop

Immediately stop giving back blows and chest thrusts if the object is coughed up or the infant begins to breathe or cough. Watch the infant, and make sure that the infant is breathing freely again. Even after the infant coughs up the object, he or she may have breathing and lung problems that will need a doctor's attention. You should also realize that chest thrusts may cause internal injuries. For these reasons, you should call the EMS system if you have not already done so. **The infant should be taken to the hospital emergency department even if he or she seems to be breathing well.**

Review Questions

Check the best answer.

3. When you are giving back blows and chest thrusts to a choking infant, the infant's head should be—
   - ☒ a. Lower than the chest.
   - ☐ b. On the same level as the chest.
   - ☐ c. Higher than the chest.

4. When you give back blows to a choking infant, where should you place your hand?
   - ☐ a. On the back of the neck
   - ☒ b. Between the shoulder blades
   - ☐ c. In the middle of the back at the level of the infant's waist

5. When you give back blows, what part of your hand should you use?
   - ☐ a. The palm
   - ☒ b. The heel
   - ☐ c. The knuckles

6. When you give chest thrusts to an infant, where should you place your fingers?
   - ☒ a. On the breastbone, one finger width below the level of the nipples
   - ☐ b. Just above the navel and well below the lower tip of the breastbone
   - ☐ c. On the navel

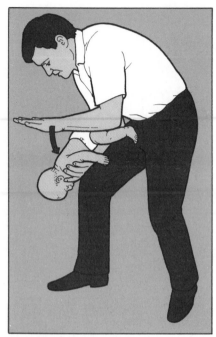

Figure 94
Give 4 Back Blows

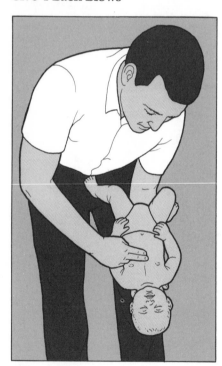

Figure 95
Give 4 Chest Thrusts

Answers

3. a. When you are giving back blows and chest thrusts to an infant, the infant's head should be **lower than the chest.**

4. b. When you give back blows to an infant, you should place your hand **between the shoulder blades.**

5. b. When you give back blows, you should use **the heel** of your hand.

6. a. When you give chest thrusts to an infant, you should place your fingers **on the breastbone, one finger width below the level of the nipples.**

First Aid for an <u>Unconscious</u> Infant With a Complete Airway Obstruction

First aid for an unconscious infant who has a complete airway obstruction begins with a primary survey. While checking the ABCs, you may find that the infant has an obstructed airway. The procedure for identifying a complete airway obstruction in an unconscious infant is given below. You should start by surveying the scene and then do a primary survey.
1. Check for unresponsiveness.
2. Shout for help.
3. Position the infant on his or her back.
4. Open the airway.
5. Look, listen, and feel for breathing.
6. Give 2 slow breaths.
7. If you are unable to breathe air into the infant, retilt the head and give 2 more breaths. You may not have tilted the infant's head into the correct position the first time.

If you still cannot breathe air into the infant, tell someone to phone the EMS system for help and do the following:
8. Give 4 back blows *(Fig. 94)* (as explained on pages 226 and 227).
9. Give 4 chest thrusts *(Fig. 95)* (as explained on pages 227 and 228).
10. Do a foreign-body check (as explained on the next page).
11. Open the airway and give 2 slow breaths.

Repeat steps 8, 9, 10, and 11 until the obstruction is cleared or EMS personnel arrive and take over.

Foreign-Body Check

To do a foreign-body check—

- Stand or kneel beside the infant's head.
- Open the infant's mouth using the hand that is nearest to the infant's feet. Put your thumb into the infant's mouth and hold both the tongue and the lower jaw between your thumb and fingers *(Fig. 96)*. Lift the jaw upward. This will bring the tongue away from the back of the throat and away from any object that may be lodged there. Look for the object, and only if you can see it, try to remove it by doing a finger sweep.

Note: To do the finger sweep, slide the little finger of your other hand into the infant's mouth. Slide your finger down along the inside of the cheek to the base of the tongue *(Fig. 97)*. Be careful not to push the object deeper into the airway. Then use a hooking action to loosen the object and move it into the mouth so that it can be removed. If you can reach the object, take it out.

Remember: Do the finger sweep only if you can see the object in the infant's throat.

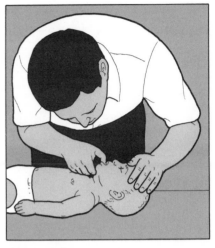

Figure 96
Foreign-Body Check

Give 2 Slow Breaths

After you do the foreign-body check, give 2 slow breaths, as follows:

- Open the airway with the head-tilt/chin-lift.
- Give 2 slow breaths.

Continue these four steps:

1. Give 4 back blows
2. Give 4 chest thrusts
3. Do a foreign-body check
4. Open the airway and give 2 slow breaths.

If your first attempts to clear the airway are unsuccessful, do not stop. The longer the infant goes without oxygen, the more the muscles of the throat will relax, making it more likely that you will be able to remove the obstruction.

If you are able to breathe air into the infant's lungs, give 2 slow breaths as you did for rescue breathing. Then check the infant's pulse. If there is no pulse, begin CPR, which you will learn in Chapter 12. If there is a pulse and the infant is not breathing on his or her own, continue rescue breathing.

If the infant starts breathing on his or her own, monitor breathing and pulse until EMS personnel arrive and take over. This means you should maintain an open airway; look, listen, and feel for breathing; and keep checking the pulse. Also, cover the infant, and keep him or her warm and as quiet as possible.

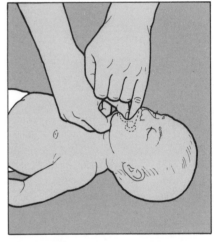

Figure 97
Finger Sweep for an Infant

Put the Steps Together

Here is the whole procedure for an unconscious infant who may have a complete airway obstruction:

1. Check for unresponsiveness.
2. Shout for help.
3. Position the infant on his or her back.
4. Open the airway.
5. Look, listen, and feel for breathing.
6. Give 2 slow breaths.
7. Retilt the head if you are unable to breathe air into the infant.
8. Give 2 slow breaths.

If you are still unable to breathe air into the infant's lungs, have someone phone the EMS system for help and—

9. Give 4 back blows.
10. Give 4 chest thrusts.
11. Do a foreign-body check.
12. Open the infant's airway and give 2 slow breaths.

Repeat steps 9, 10, 11, and 12 in the same order until the obstruction is cleared or EMS personnel arrive and take over. If you succeed in removing the object, open the airway and give 2 slow breaths. Then check for a pulse. If there is no pulse, begin CPR. If there is a pulse, check for breathing. If the infant is not breathing on his or her own, continue rescue breathing.

Review Questions

Check the best answer.

7. An unconscious infant is not breathing. If you cannot breathe air into the infant's lungs on the first try, what should you do next?
   - ☒ a. Retilt the head and give 2 slow breaths.
   - ☐ b. Do a foreign-body check.
   - ☐ c. Give back blows and chest thrusts.

8. For an unconscious infant who has a complete airway obstruction, how many back blows and chest thrusts should you do before doing a foreign-body check?
   - ☐ a. 4 back blows and 2 chest thrusts
   - ☐ b. 6 back blows and 4 chest thrusts
   - ☒ c. 4 back blows and 4 chest thrusts

9. After removing an object from an infant's mouth, you give 2 slow breaths and see the infant's chest rise and fall. What should you do next?
   - ☐ a. Open the airway.
   - ☒ b. Check the pulse.
   - ☐ c. Phone the EMS system for help.

10. When should you do a finger sweep on an infant?
   - ☒ a. When you can see the object in the infant's throat
   - ☐ b. When the second set of 2 slow breaths will not go into the infant's lungs
   - ☐ c. When you think the infant has swallowed an object

Answers

7. **a.** **Retilt the head and give 2 slow breaths** if you cannot breathe air into an unconscious infant who is not breathing.

8. **c.** You should give **4 back blows and 4 chest thrusts** before doing a foreign-body check.

9. **b.** If you are able to breathe air into the infant, the next thing you should do is **check the pulse.**

10. **a.** You should do a finger sweep on an infant **when you can see the object in the infant's throat.**

First Aid for Choking When a Conscious Infant Becomes Unconscious

If an infant becomes unconscious while you are giving first aid for choking, you should shout for help. Have someone phone the EMS system for help if it hasn't already been done. Place the infant on a firm, flat surface. Then—

1. Do a foreign-body check.
2. Open the airway and give 2 slow breaths.
3. Give 4 back blows.
4. Give 4 chest thrusts.

Repeat these four steps until the obstruction is cleared or EMS personnel arrive and take over.

If you are able to breathe air into the infant's lungs, give 2 slow breaths as you did for rescue breathing. Then check the pulse. If the infant has no pulse, then you must begin CPR. If there is a pulse and the infant is not breathing on his or her own, continue doing rescue breathing.

If the infant starts breathing on his or her own, monitor breathing and pulse until EMS personnel arrive and take over. This means you should maintain an open airway; look, listen, and feel for the infant's breathing; and keep checking the pulse. Also, cover the infant, and keep him or her warm and as quiet as possible.

Practice Session: First Aid for an Infant Who Is Choking

During this two-part practice session, you and a partner will practice only on a manikin.

You will learn two separate skills: first aid for a **conscious** infant with a complete airway obstruction, and first aid for an **unconscious** infant with a complete airway obstruction.

1. You will practice first aid for a conscious infant with a complete airway obstruction.

    Before you start practicing, carefully read the skill sheet on pages 236 through 240. If you don't remember how to use the checklist, read pages 44 through 46.

2. You will practice first aid for an unconscious infant with a complete airway obstruction.

    Before you start practicing, carefully read the skill sheet on pages 241 through 250. If you don't remember how to use the checklist, read pages 44 through 46. You will practice this skill on a manikin. Do not touch the manikin's lips or inside the mouth with your fingers.

    Before you practice on the manikin, clean its face and the inside of its mouth. Directions for doing this are given in the section called "Some Health Precautions and Guidelines to Follow During This Course" on page 3 of this workbook. Clean the manikin's face and mouth before each person in your group practices.

*Skill Sheet: First Aid for a Conscious Infant With a
Complete Airway Obstruction*

Partner Check

Instructor Check

☐ ☑ **Determine If Infant Is Choking**

Determine if infant can cry, cough, or breathe.

Partner/Instructor says, "Infant cannot cry, cough, or breathe."

Rescuer shouts, "Help!"

☐ ☑ **Phone the EMS System for Help**

Tell someone to call for an ambulance.

Rescuer says, "Infant choking,
call _____."
(*Local emergency number or Operator*)

☐ ☑ **Give 4 Back Blows**

Grasp infant's jaw with your thumb and fingers.

Slide your hand behind infant's shoulder blade closest to you
so that your fingers support back of infant's head and neck.

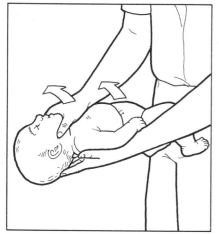

Turn infant over so that infant is facedown on your forearm.

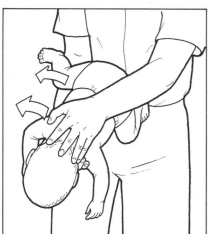

Support infant's head and neck with your hand by firmly holding the jaw between your thumb and fingers.

Lower your forearm onto your thigh. Infant's head should be lower than the chest.

Give 4 back blows forcefully between infant's shoulder blades with heel of your other hand.

Each back blow should be a separate and distinct attempt to dislodge object.

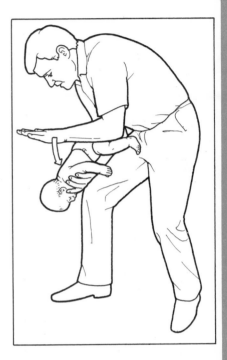

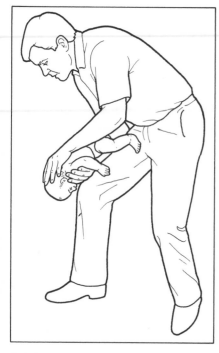

☐ ☑ **Give 4 Chest Thrusts**

Turn infant onto back:

> Place your free hand and forearm along infant's head and back so that infant is sandwiched between your two hands and forearms.

> Support back of infant's head and neck with your fingers.

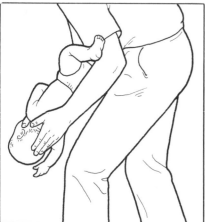

Turn infant onto his or her back, keeping head and body straight.

Lower your forearm onto your thigh.

Keep infant's head lower than his or her chest.

Locate position for chest thrusts:
  Imagine a line running across infant's chest connecting
  nipples.

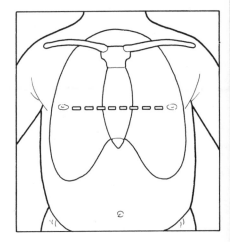

Place pad of ring finger on breastbone just below this
imaginary line.

Place pads of next two fingers on breastbone beside the ring
finger.

Pads of fingers should lie along length of breastbone.

Raise ring finger.

If you feel the notch at the end of the breastbone, move your
fingers up a little bit.

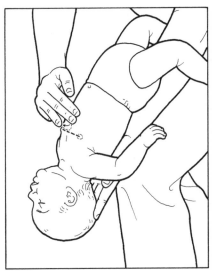

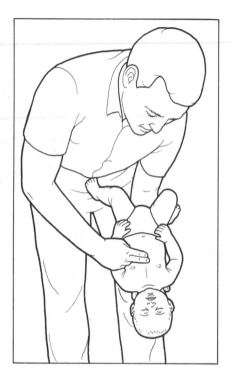

Partner Check
Instructor Check

Give 4 chest thrusts:

Using pads of two fingers, compress breastbone ½ to 1 inch (1.3 to 2.5 centimeters), 4 times.

Compress down and up smoothly, keeping your fingers in contact with chest at all times.

Each thrust should be a separate and distinct attempt to dislodge the object.

☐ ☑ **Repeat Back Blows and Chest Thrusts**
Continue giving back blows and chest thrusts until obstruction is cleared or infant becomes unconscious.

Final Instructor Check *MEL*

Skill Sheet: First Aid for an Unconscious Infant With a Complete Airway Obstruction

You find an infant lying unusually still, and you suspect that something may be wrong. You should survey the scene to see if it is safe and to get some idea of what happened. Then do a primary survey by checking the ABCs.

Remember: **Do not do finger sweeps on a manikin. Do not touch the manikin's lips or inside the mouth with your fingers.**

Partner Check
Instructor Check

☐ ☐ **Check for Unresponsiveness**

Tap or gently shake infant's shoulder.

Partner/Instructor says, "Unconscious."

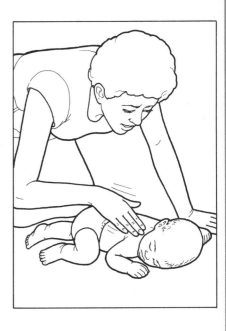

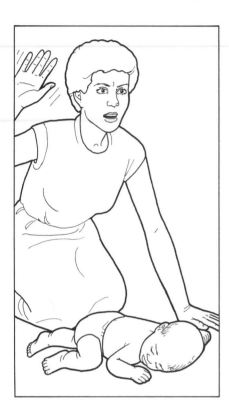

Rescuer repeats, "Unconscious."
Rescuer shouts, "Help!"

Position the Infant

Roll infant onto back, if necessary.

Stand or kneel facing infant.

Straighten infant's legs, if necessary, and move infant's arm closest to you above infant's head.

Lean over infant and place one hand on infant's shoulder and other hand on infant's hip.

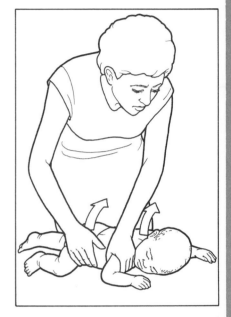

Roll infant toward you as a single unit. As you roll infant, move your hand from infant's shoulder to support back of head and neck.

Place infant's arm closest to you alongside infant's body.

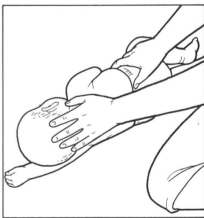

Partner Check
Instructor Check

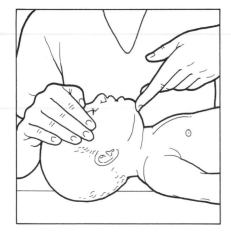

☐ ☑ **Open the Airway** (Use head-tilt/chin-lift)

Place your hand— the one nearest the infant's head— on infant's forehead.

Place fingers of other hand under bony part of lower jaw at the chin.

Tilt head gently back into the neutral position and lift chin. Avoid closing infant's mouth completely. Avoid pushing on the soft parts under the chin.

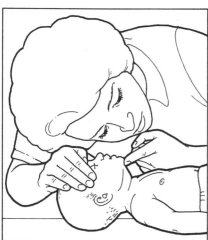

☐ ☑ **Check for Breathlessness**

Maintain open airway with head-tilt/chin-lift.

Place your ear over infant's mouth and nose.

Look at chest and abdomen; listen and feel for breathing for 3 to 5 seconds.

Partner/Instructor says, "No breathing."

Rescuer repeats, "No breathing."

☐ ☑ **Give 2 Slow Breaths**

Maintain open airway with head-tilt/chin-lift.

Open your mouth wide, take a breath, and seal your lips tightly around infant's mouth and nose.

Give 2 slow breaths at the rate of 1 to 1½ seconds per breath. Pause in between each breath for you to take a breath.

Partner/Instructor says, "Unable to breathe air into infant."

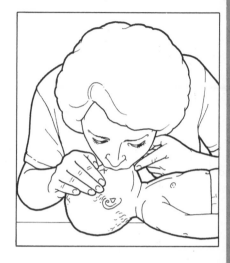

☐ ☑ **Retilt Infant's Head and Give 2 Slow Breaths**

Retilt infant's head and lift chin. Avoid closing infant's mouth completely. Avoid pushing on the soft parts under the chin.

Open your mouth wide, take a breath, and seal your lips tightly around infant's mouth and nose.

Give 2 slow breaths at the rate of 1 to 1½ seconds per breath. Pause in between each breath for you to take a breath.

Partner/Instructor says, "Still unable to breathe air into infant."

Rescuer says, "Airway obstructed."

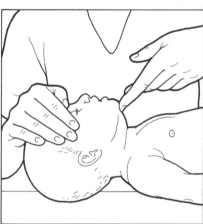

☐ ☑ **Phone the EMS System for Help**

Tell someone to call for an ambulance.

Rescuer says, "Infant's airway obstructed, call _____."
(*Local emergency number or Operator*)

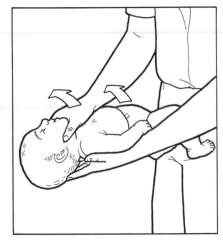

Partner Check
Instructor Check

☐ ☐ **Give 4 Back Blows**

Grasp infant's jaw with your thumb and fingers.

Slide your hand behind infant's shoulder blade closest to you so that your fingers support the back of infant's head and neck.

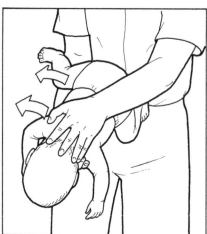

Turn infant over so that infant is facedown on your forearm.

Support infant's head and neck with your hand by firmly holding the jaw between your thumb and fingers.

Lower your forearm onto your thigh. Infant's head should be lower than the chest.

Give 4 back blows forcefully between infant's shoulder blades with heel of your other hand.

Each back blow should be a separate and distinct attempt to dislodge object.

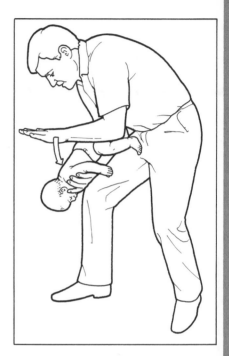

☐ ☑ **Give 4 Chest Thrusts**
Turn infant onto back:
  Place your free hand and forearm along infant's head and back so that infant is sandwiched between your two hands and forearms.

  Support back of infant's head and neck with your fingers.

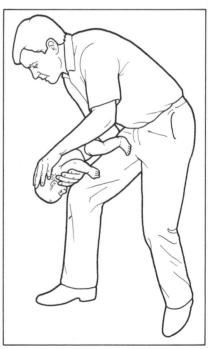

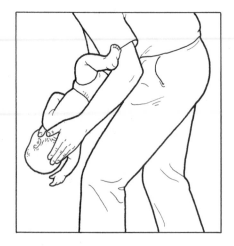

Turn infant onto his or her back keeping head and body straight.

Lower your forearm onto your thigh.

Keep infant's head lower than his or her chest.

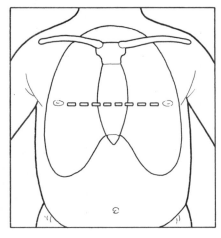

Locate position for chest thrusts:
  Imagine a line running across infant's chest connecting nipples.

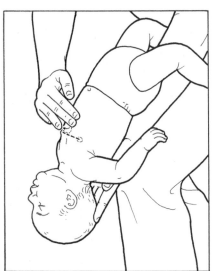

Place pad of ring finger on breastbone just below this imaginary line.

Place pads of next two fingers on breastbone beside the ring finger.

Pads of fingers should lie along length of breastbone.

Raise ring finger.

If you feel the notch at the end of the breastbone, move your fingers up a little bit.

Partner Check
Instructor Check

Give 4 chest thrusts:

Using pads of two fingers, compress breastbone ½ to 1 inch (1.3 to 2.5 centimeters), 4 times.

Compress down and up smoothly, keeping your fingers in contact with chest at all times.

Each thrust should be a separate and distinct attempt to dislodge the object.

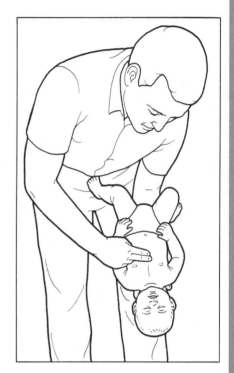

☐ ☑ **Foreign-Body Check**

With infant's face up, open his or her mouth by grasping both tongue and lower jaw between thumb and fingers of hand nearest infant's legs. Lift jaw.

Look inside mouth for object. If object is visible, attempt to remove it.

Partner/Instructor says, "No object seen."

Rescuer repeats, "No object seen."

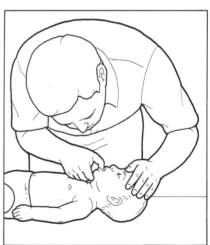

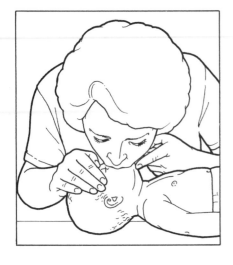

Partner Check
Instructor Check

☐ ☐ **Give 2 Slow Breaths**

Maintain open airway with head-tilt/chin-lift.

Open your mouth wide, take a breath, and seal your lips tightly around infant's mouth and nose.

Give 2 slow breaths at the rate of 1 to 1½ seconds per breath. Pause in between each breath for you to take a breath. Partner/Instructor says, "Airway still obstructed."

☐ ☐ **Repeat Sequence**

Give 4 back blows.

Give 4 chest thrusts.

Do foreign-body check.

Give 2 slow breaths.

☐ ☐ **What to Do Next**

While the rescuer is repeating the sequence of back blows, chest thrusts, foreign-body check, and rescue breaths, the partner should read one of the following statements:

1. Rescuer can breathe into infant's lungs after doing foreign-body check.
2. After foreign-body check, object is removed with finger sweep.
3. Object is expelled during chest thrusts.

Based on this information, the rescuer should decide what to do next and continue giving the right care.

Final Instructor Check _MER_

12 *What to Do When an Infant's Heart Stops (CPR)*

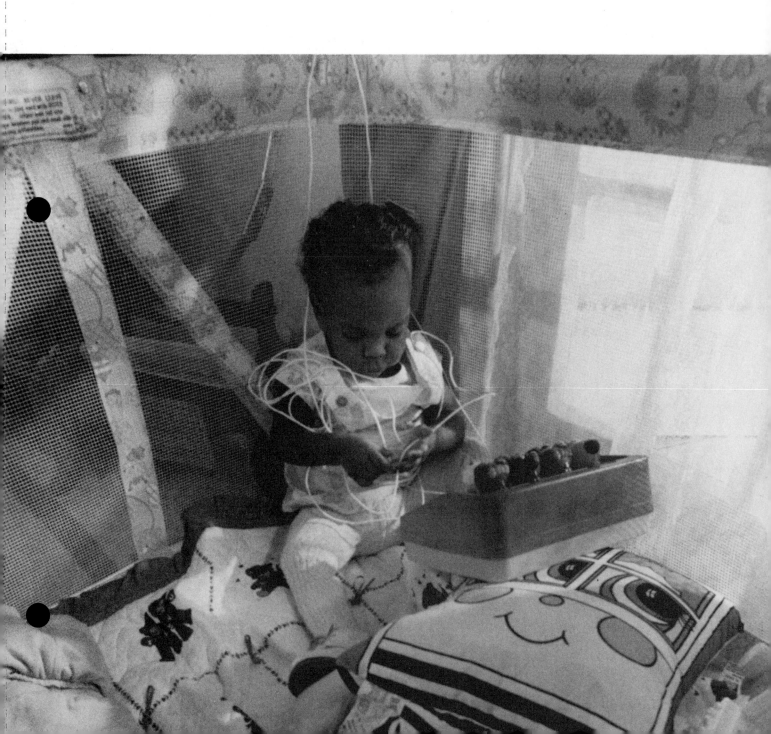

In Chapter 9, you learned how to give CPR to a child age one through eight. In this chapter, you will learn how to give CPR to an infant newborn to age one. When an infant's heart stops, his or her survival depends on how quickly CPR is started and how quickly he or she receives advanced emergency medical care.

In this chapter, you will learn what to do for an infant whose heart has stopped beating. You will learn how to keep oxygen-carrying blood moving through the infant's body.

Objectives

By the time you finish reading this chapter, you should be able to do the following:

1. *Describe the early signals of a cardiac emergency.*
2. *Recognize when an infant needs CPR.*
3. *Explain why it is important to check the infant's brachial pulse before you start CPR.*
4. *Describe how to give CPR to an infant.*
5. *Describe when you should check for the return of the infant's pulse after you start CPR.*
6. *List four conditions when a rescuer may stop CPR.*

Cardiac Emergencies in Infants

The most common cause of cardiac emergencies in infants is sudden infant death syndrome (SIDS). Other common causes include injuries resulting from motor vehicle accidents, poisoning, airway obstruction, suffocation, smoke inhalation, burns, and near-drowning. A cardiac emergency can also be the result of a medical condition or illness such as severe croup, or respiratory infections such as epiglottitis or severe bronchiolitis.

Except for SIDS, most cardiac emergencies in infants are preventable. One way to prevent cardiac emergencies is to prevent infants from being injured. In Chapter 6, you read about how you can reduce the risk of injury. Second, it is important to make sure infants receive proper medical care. A third preventive measure is learning to recognize the early signals of a respiratory emergency since a cardiac emergency may result from a respiratory emergency. These signals may include any of the following:

- Agitation
- Drowsiness
- Change in skin color (to pale, blue, or gray)
- Increased difficulty in breathing
- Increased heart and breathing rates

In this chapter, you will learn how to give first aid to an infant who has suffered a cardiac emergency. When a cardiac emergency does happen, you should immediately begin first aid as described below.

How to Give CPR to an Infant

To find out if an infant needs CPR, begin with a primary survey to check the ABCs. You should—

1. Check for unresponsiveness.
2. Shout for help.
3. Position the infant on his or her back.
4. Open the airway.
5. Look, listen, and feel for breathing.
6. If the infant is not breathing, give 2 slow breaths.
7. Check the brachial pulse.
8. Have someone phone the EMS system for help.

If the infant has no pulse, begin CPR. **It is important to check the infant's brachial pulse for 5 to 10 seconds before you start CPR because it is dangerous to do chest compressions if the infant's heart is beating.**

Locating the Compression Position

For chest compressions to work, the infant must be lying flat on his or her back on a firm, flat surface. The infant's head must be on the same level as the heart.

To give effective compressions, your hands and body must be in the correct position. Do the following:

- Lay the infant on a firm, flat surface.
- Stand or kneel facing the infant from the side.
- Use your hand—the one nearest the infant's head—to keep the infant's head in the neutral position.
- Use your other hand—the one nearest the infant's legs—to find the correct place to give compressions. Imagine a line running across the chest between the infant's nipples (*Fig. 98*). Put the pad of your index finger on the breastbone just below this imaginary line.
- Put the pads of two fingers next to your index finger on the breastbone.
- Raise the index finger (*Fig. 99*). If you feel the notch at the end of the breastbone, move your fingers slightly toward the head.

Having your fingers in the correct position will lessen the chance of fracturing the ribs on either side of the infant's breastbone.

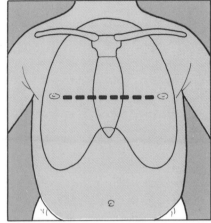

Figure 98
Imaginary Line Between Nipples

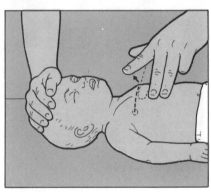

Figure 99
Position for Giving Compressions

Review Questions

Check the best answer(s).

1. On which of the following surfaces should you give CPR to an infant? (Check all that apply.)
   - ☐ a. Crib
   - ☐ b. Couch
   - ☒ c. Floor
   - ☒ d. Table

2. Where should your fingers be when you give chest compressions to an infant?
   - ☒ a. On the breastbone one finger width below an imaginary line connecting the infant's nipples
   - ☐ b. At the top of the breastbone where it joins the collar bones
   - ☐ c. At the lower tip of the breastbone

Answers

1. When you give CPR to an infant, the infant should be on a firm, flat surface such as—
   c. The **floor**, or
   d. A **table**.

2. a. When you give chest compressions to an infant, your fingers should be **on the breastbone one finger width below an imaginary line connecting the infant's nipples.**

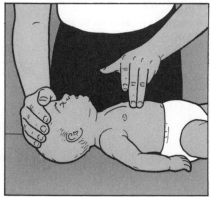

Figure 100
Give Chest Compressions

Compression Technique
This is how you give chest compressions to an infant:
1. When you compress, use only the fingers that are on the infant's breastbone (*Fig. 100*). You will **not** use the heel of your hand as you did when you practiced CPR for a child. When you compress, push straight down. If you don't push straight down, your compressions will not be effective.

2. Each compression should push the infant's breastbone down from ½ to 1 inch (1.3 to 2.5 centimeters) (*Fig. 101*). Your elbow should be bent, and the down-and-up movement of your compression should be smooth, not jerky. Keep a steady down-and-up rhythm, and do not pause between compressions. Half the time should be spent pushing down, and half the time should be spent coming up. When you are coming up, release pressure on the infant's chest completely, but don't lift your fingers off the infant's chest. Keep your fingers in the compression position. Use your other hand to keep the airway open by holding the infant's head in the neutral position.

3. Give compressions at the rate of at least 100 compressions per minute.

4. Take note of where your fingers are resting on the breastbone. When you take your hand off the infant's chest, put your fingers back in the same place before you start compressions again.

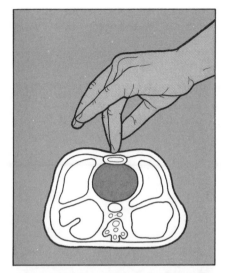

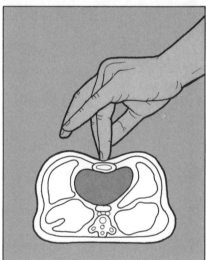

Figure 101
Compress Chest ½ to 1 Inch

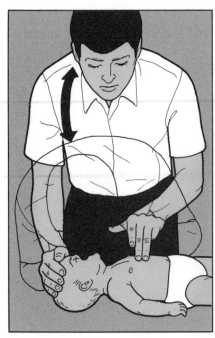

Figure 102
5 Compressions, Then 1 Breath

Compression/Breathing Cycles

When you give CPR, do cycles of 5 compressions and 1 breath (*Fig. 102*). In each cycle, give 5 compressions with the fingers of one hand while you keep your other hand on the infant's forehead to keep the head in the neutral position. Then give 1 breath. If the chest does not rise when you breathe into the infant, remove your fingers from the chest and lift the chin to open the airway. Then return your fingers to the infant's breastbone to continue compression/breathing cycles.

Put the Steps Together

Here are the steps you should follow when you give CPR to an infant:

1. Check for unresponsiveness.

2. Shout for help.

3. Position the infant on his or her back.

4. Open the airway.

5. Look, listen, and feel for breathing (3 to 5 seconds).

6. If the infant is not breathing, give 2 slow breaths.

7. Check the infant's brachial pulse for heartbeat (5 to 10 seconds).

8. Tell someone to phone the EMS system for help.

9. If there is no pulse, find the correct finger position to give chest compressions.

10. Give 5 compressions without stopping, at a rate of at least 100 per minute. Count out loud very quickly, "One, two, three, four, five." Remember to keep your other hand on the infant's forehead, keeping the head in the neutral position.

11. When you stop compressions, keep your hand on the chest. Use your other hand to hold the infant's head in the neutral position. Give 1 slow breath to the infant, covering the infant's nose and mouth with your mouth. The breath should take about 1 to 1½ seconds.

12. Keep repeating—5 compressions, 1 breath, 5 compressions, 1 breath, and so on. The complete cycle of 5 compressions and 1 breath should take from 3 to 5 seconds.

13. Recheck pulse. After you do about 10 cycles (or about 1 minute) of continuous CPR, check to see if the infant has a pulse. Do this after you give the breath at the end of the 10th cycle of 5 compressions and 1 breath. Check the brachial pulse for 5 seconds with the hand that was giving compressions. If there is no pulse, return your hand to the infant's chest, give 1 breath, and continue CPR. Repeat the pulse check every few minutes.

If you do find a pulse, then check for breathing for 3 to 5 seconds. If the infant is breathing, keep the airway open and monitor breathing and pulse closely. This means that you should look, listen, and feel for breathing. Check the pulse once every minute. Cover the infant, and keep the infant warm and as quiet as possible. If the infant is not breathing, give rescue breathing and keep checking the pulse.

14. Continue CPR until one of these things happens:
    - The heart starts beating again.
    - A second rescuer trained in CPR takes over for you.
    - EMS personnel arrive and take over.
    - You are too exhausted to continue.

Review Questions

Check the best answer.

3. How far should you compress the chest of an infant?
   - ☐ a. ½ to 1 inch (1.3 to 2.5 centimeters)
   - ☐ b. 1 to 1½ inches (2.5 to 3.8 centimeters)
   - ☐ c. 1½ to 2 inches (3.8 to 5 centimeters)

4. When you give CPR to an infant, at what rate should you give chest compressions?
   - ☐ a. 50 to 60 times per minute
   - ☐ b. 60 to 80 times per minute
   - ☐ c. At least 100 times per minute

5. When you give CPR to an infant, what is the ratio of compressions to breaths?
   - ☐ a. 5 compressions, then 1 breath
   - ☐ b. 10 compressions, then 2 breaths
   - ☐ c. 15 compressions, then 2 breaths

6. After starting CPR on an infant, how often should you check for the return of pulse?
   - ☐ a. After 5 minutes and every 5 to 6 minutes thereafter
   - ☐ b. After 2 minutes and every 4 to 5 minutes thereafter
   - ☐ c. After 1 minute and every few minutes thereafter

Answers

3. **a.** You should compress the chest of an infant ½ **to 1 inch (1.3 to 2.5 centimeters).**

4. **c.** When you give CPR to an infant, you should compress the chest at the rate of **at least 100 times per minute.**

5. **a.** When you give CPR to an infant, the ratio is **5 compressions, then 1 breath.**

6. **c.** After starting CPR on an infant, you should check for the return of pulse **after 1 minute and every few minutes thereafter.**

More About CPR for an Infant

If No One Comes When You Shout for Help

One of the first things you do when you discover an unresponsive infant is to shout for help. You do this to attract the attention of someone nearby who can phone the EMS system for help. But what if no one responds to your shouts for help? You should do CPR for at least 1 minute. During this minute you should continue to shout for help. You should also use this minute to plan how to make the call yourself.

If no one has answered your shouts for help by the end of 1 minute of CPR, you should get to a phone as quickly as you can and call the EMS system. If possible, you should bring the phone to the area where the infant is or carry the infant with you to the phone. Then begin CPR again.

If a Second Trained Rescuer Is at the Scene

If another rescuer trained in CPR is at the scene, this person should do two things: first, phone the EMS system for help if this has not been done; second, take over CPR when the first rescuer is tired. Here are the steps for entry of the second rescuer:

- The second person should identify himself or herself as a CPR-trained rescuer who is willing to help.
- If the EMS system has been called and if the first rescuer is tired and asks for help, then—

   1. The first rescuer should stop CPR after the next breath.

   2. The second rescuer should stand or kneel beside the infant opposite the first rescuer, tilt the head into the neutral position, and feel for the brachial pulse for 5 seconds.

   3. If there is no pulse, the second rescuer should give 1 breath and continue CPR.

   4. The first rescuer should then check the adequacy of the second rescuer's breaths and chest compressions. This is done by watching the infant's chest rise and fall during rescue breathing, and by feeling the brachial pulse for an artificial pulse during chest compressions. This artificial pulse will tell you that blood is moving through the body.

Practice Session: CPR for an Infant

During this practice session, you and a partner will practice only on a manikin.

Before you start practicing, carefully read the skill sheet on pages 260 through 267. If you don't remember how to use the checklist, read pages 44 through 46.

Before you practice on the manikin, clean its face and the inside of its mouth. Directions for doing this are given in the section called "Some Health Precautions and Guidelines to Follow During This Course" on page 3 of this workbook. Clean the manikin's face and mouth before each person in your group practices.

Skill Sheet: CPR for an Infant

You find an infant lying unusually still, and you suspect that something may be wrong. You should survey the scene to see if it is safe and to get some idea of what happened. Then do a primary survey by checking the ABCs.

Partner Check
Instructor Check

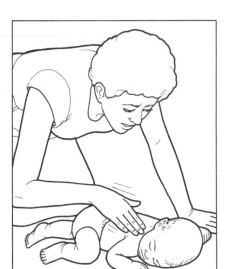

☐ ☐ **Check for Unresponsiveness**

Tap or gently shake infant's shoulder.

Partner/Instructor says, "Unconscious."

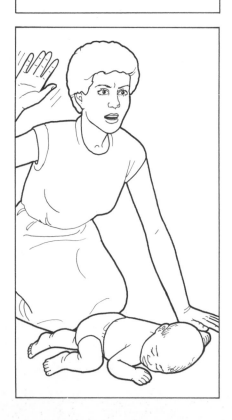

Rescuer repeats, "Unconscious."

Rescuer shouts, "Help!"

Position the Infant

Roll infant onto back, if necessary.

Stand or kneel facing infant.

Straighten infant's legs, if necessary, and move infant's arm closest to you above infant's head.

Lean over infant and place one hand on infant's shoulder and other hand on infant's hip.

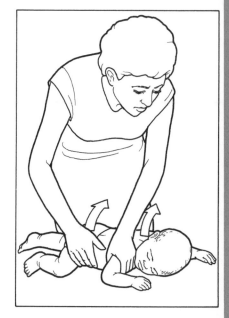

Roll infant toward you as a single unit. As you roll infant, move your hand from infant's shoulder to support back of head and neck.

Place infant's arm closest to you alongside infant's body.

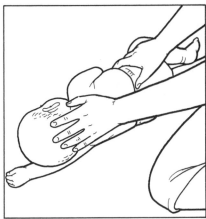

Practice Session: CPR for an Infant

Partner Check
Instructor Check

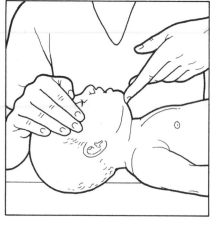

☐ ☐ **Open the Airway** (Use head-tilt/chin-lift.)

Place your hand—the one nearest infant's head—on infant's forehead.

Place fingers of other hand under bony part of lower jaw at the chin.

Tilt head gently back into neutral position and lift chin. Avoid closing infant's mouth completely. Avoid pushing on the soft parts under the chin.

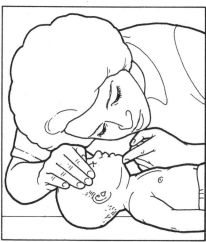

☐ ☐ **Check for Breathlessness**

Maintain open airway with head-tilt/chin-lift.

Place your ear over infant's mouth and nose.

Look at chest and abdomen; listen and feel for breathing for 3 to 5 seconds.

Partner/Instructor says, "No breathing."

Rescuer repeats, "No breathing."

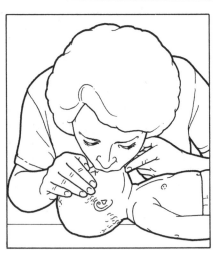

☐ ☐ **Give 2 Slow Breaths**

Maintain open airway with head-tilt/chin-lift.

Open your mouth wide, take a breath, and seal your lips tightly around infant's mouth and nose.

Give 2 slow breaths at the rate of 1 to 1½ seconds per breath. Pause in between each breath for you to take a breath.

Look for the chest to rise and fall; listen and feel for escaping air.

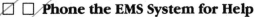
Partner Check
Instructor Check

☐ ☐ **Check for Pulse**

Maintain head-tilt with one hand on forehead.

Place thumb of other hand on outside of infant's upper arm closest to you. Your thumb should be halfway between the shoulder and elbow. Press gently with your index and middle fingers on inside of arm.

Feel for brachial pulse for 5 to 10 seconds.

Partner/Instructor says, "No breathing and no pulse."

Rescuer repeats, "No breathing, and no pulse."

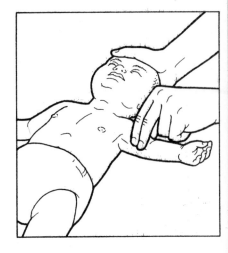

☑ ☐ **Phone the EMS System for Help**

Tell someone to call for an ambulance.

Rescuer says, "Infant not breathing, has no pulse, call _____."
(Local emergency number or Operator)

☑ ☐ **Locate Compression Position**

Stand or kneel facing infant.

Maintain head-tilt with hand on forehead.

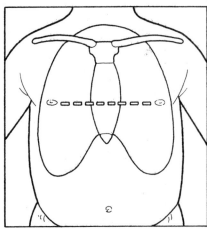

Imagine a line running across the chest connecting the nipples.

Place pad of your index finger on breastbone just below this imaginary line.

Place pads of two fingers next to your index finger on breastbone.

Pads of fingers should lie along length of breastbone.

Raise your index finger.

If you feel notch at end of breastbone, move your fingers up a little bit.

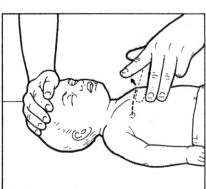

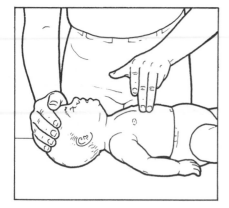

Partner Check Instructor Check

□ □ **Give 5 Compressions**

Compress breastbone ½ to 1 inch (1.3 to 2.5 centimeters) at a rate of at least 100 compressions per minute (5 compressions should take 3 seconds or less).

Count aloud very quickly "One, two, three, four, five."

Compress down and up smoothly, keeping hand contact with chest at all times.

Maintain head-tilt with hand on forehead

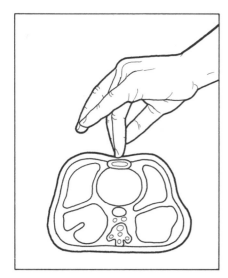

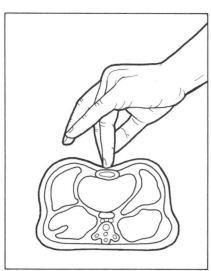

☐ ☐ **Give 1 Slow Breath**

Stop compressions. Keep fingers in position.

Maintain head-tilt with hand on forehead.

Open your mouth wide, take a breath, and seal your lips tightly around infant's mouth and nose.

Give 1 slow breath (lasting 1 to 1½ seconds).

Look for the chest to rise and fall; listen and feel for escaping air.

If chest does not rise, use hand on chest to perform chin- lift.

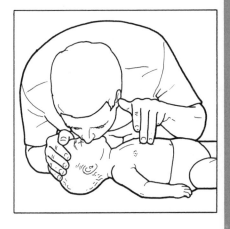

☐ ☐ **Do Compression/Breathing Cycles**

Keep head tilted with one hand on forehead.

Do 10 cycles of 5 compressions and 1 breath.

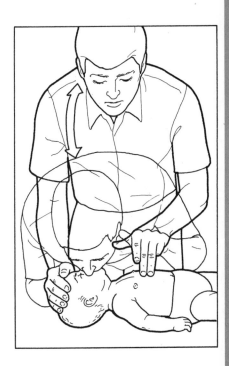

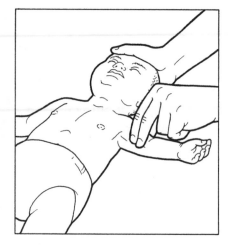

Partner Check

Instructor Check

☑ ☐ **Recheck Pulse**

Maintain head-tilt with one hand on forehead.

Feel for brachial pulse for 5 seconds with hand that was giving compressions.

Partner/Instructor says, "No pulse."

Rescuer repeats, "No pulse."

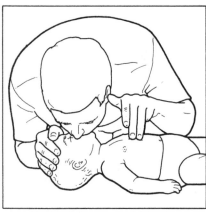

☑ ☐ **Give 1 Slow Breath**

Return hand to chest. Locate compression point.

Maintain head-tilt with hand on forehead.

Open your mouth wide, take a breath, and seal your lips tightly around infant's mouth and nose.

Give 1 slow breath (lasting 1 to 1½ seconds per breath).

Look for the chest to rise and fall; listen and feel for escaping air.

If chest does not rise, use hand on chest to perform chin-lift.

Partner Check
Instructor Check

☐ ☐ **Continue Compression Breathing Cycles**

Continue cycles of 5 compressions and 1 breath.

Recheck pulse every few minutes.

☐ ☐ **What to Do Next**

When the rescuer stops to check pulse, the partner should read one of the following statements:

1. Infant has a pulse.

2. Infant does not have a pulse.

Based on this information, the rescuer should decide what to do next and continue giving the right care.

Final Instructor Check

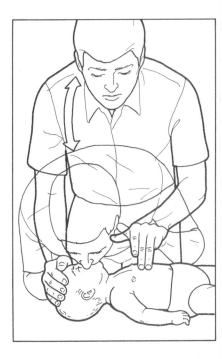

Review Questions for Unit Two

Directions

This section will help you review what you have learned in this unit. You will be presented with a number of situations that you may find in real life. The questions will ask you what you would do if you came across those situations. Choose the correct answer or fill in the blanks. The correct answers follow each group of questions.

Review Question: Rescue Breathing for a Child

A seven-year-old boy has just been pulled out of a swimming pool. You run over to him and check for unresponsiveness. He is unconscious.

When you check the ABCs, you find that he is not breathing but does have a pulse. Someone calls the EMS system while you begin rescue breathing.

1. How often should you give rescue breaths to a child?
   - ☐ a. Give 1 breath every second.
   - ☒ b. Give 1 breath every 4 seconds.
   - ☐ c. Give 1 breath every 8 seconds.

You recheck the pulse after 1 minute of rescue breathing, and find that the child still has a pulse.

2. What should you do next?
   - ☒ a. Check for breathing for 3 to 5 seconds.
   - ☐ b. Continue rescue breathing.
   - ☐ c. Give 2 slow breaths.

3. If the child starts to breathe on his own, what should you do until EMS personnel arrive?
   - ☐ a. Leave the child alone.
   - ☒ b. Monitor breathing and pulse closely.
   - ☐ c. Continue giving 1 rescue breath every 4 seconds.

Child

Answers

1. **b.** For a child, you should **give 1 breath every 4 seconds.**
2. **a.** You should **check for breathing for 3 to 5 seconds.**
3. **b.** You should **monitor breathing and pulse closely** until EMS personnel arrive if the child starts to breathe on his own.

Review Question: First Aid for a Conscious Child With an Obstructed Airway

Your five-year-old nephew is eating a piece of hard candy and talking to you at the same time. Suddenly he stops talking and seems to gag. You begin first aid by asking, "Are you choking?" but he cannot speak and grabs his throat. You shout for help and have someone phone the EMS system for help.

1. For a conscious child who is choking you—
- ☐ a. Give rescue breaths.
- ☒ b. Give abdominal thrusts.
- ☐ c. Do CPR.

Chila

Answers

1. b. You **give abdominal thrusts** to a conscious child who is choking.

Review Question: First Aid for an Unconscious Child With an Obstructed Airway

You see your neighbor's child playing on her swing and eating a snack. A few minutes later, you see her lying on the ground. You begin a primary survey by checking for unresponsiveness. She is unconscious.

1. What should you do next?
   - ☒ a. Open the airway.
   - ☐ b. Check for a pulse.
   - ☐ c. Call the EMS system.

The child is not breathing. When you give 2 slow breaths, the air will not go in.

2. What should you do now?
   - ☐ a. Do a foreign-body check.
   - ☒ b. Retilt the head and give 2 slow breaths.
   - ☐ c. Begin CPR.

You realize that the child has an obstructed airway. You tell someone to phone the EMS system for help, and then you give abdominal thrusts.

3. How many abdominal thrusts should you give before you do a foreign-body check?
   - ☐ a. 1 or 2
   - ☒ b. 6 to 10
   - ☐ c. 15 to 20

4. After doing the foreign-body check, you should give
   _____2_____ slow breaths.

After repeating the sequence of abdominal thrusts, foreign-body check, and 2 slow breaths, you are able to breathe air into the child.

5. What should you do now?
   - ☐ a. Give rescue breaths.
   - ☐ b. Keep on giving abdominal thrusts.
   - ☒ c. Check the pulse.

Child

Answers

1. a. If you find that a child is unconscious, you should **open the airway**.

2. b. You should **retilt the head and give 2 slow breaths** if air will not go into the child's lungs.

3. b. You should give **6 to 10** abdominal thrusts before you do a foreign-body check.

4. You should give **2** slow breaths after doing the foreign-body check.

5. c. You should **check the pulse** if you are able to breathe into the child after doing a foreign-body check.

Review Question: CPR for a Child

A three-year-old has been playing in the garage. You find her lying motionless on the ground next to some exposed electric wires. You begin a primary survey. The girl is unconscious. You open the airway, and give 2 slow breaths. Then you check the pulse.

1. Where should you check the pulse?
   - [ ] a. At the wrist
   - [ ] b. On the upper arm
   - [x] c. At the side of the neck

There is no pulse. You send someone to phone for an ambulance and begin CPR.

2. When you give CPR to a child, what is the ratio of compressions to breaths?
   - [x] a. 5 compressions to 1 breath
   - [ ] b. 5 compressions to 5 breaths
   - [ ] c. 10 compressions to 2 breaths

3. At what rate should you give chest compressions when giving CPR to a child?
   - [ ] a. 50 to 60 compressions per minute
   - [x] b. 80 to 100 compressions per minute
   - [ ] c. 110 to 120 compressions per minute

4. After starting CPR, how often should you check for the return of a pulse?
   - [ ] a. After 5 minutes and every 5 to 6 minutes thereafter
   - [ ] b. After 2 minutes and every 4 to 5 minutes thereafter
   - [x] c. After 1 minute and every few minutes thereafter

5. You continue CPR until one of four things happens:
   a. The heart starts _beating_ again.
   b. A second rescuer trained in _CPR_ takes over for you.
   c. _EMS_ personnel arrive and take over.
   d. You are too exhausted to continue.

Child

Answers

1. **c.** You should check a child's pulse **at the side of the neck**.

2. **a.** When you give CPR to a child, the ratio is **5 compressions to 1 breath**.

3. **b.** You should give chest compressions to a child at the rate of **80 to 100 compressions per minute.**

4. **c.** After starting CPR, you should check for the return of a pulse **after 1 minute and every few minutes thereafter.**

5. You continue CPR until—
   a. The heart starts **beating** again.
   b. A second rescuer trained in **CPR** takes over for you.
   c. **EMS** personnel arrive and take over.
   d. You are too exhausted to continue.

Review Question: Rescue Breathing for an Infant

You hear your neighbor shouting "Help." When you get to her, she says she found her infant lying in the crib with a big stuffed toy over her face. The infant is not moving or making any noise. You tap the infant's shoulder to check for unresponsiveness and find that she is unconscious. You continue a primary survey.

1. Fill in the blanks in the following statements.

   A—Airway   You open the airway by doing the head-tilt/_Chin_ lift. The infant's head should be tilted into the **neutral** position.

   B—Breathing   When you check for breathing, you look, _listen_, and feel for breathing.

   C—Circulation   You check the infant's pulse by pressing gently against the inside of the upper _arm_.

The infant is not breathing but has a pulse. You tell your neighbor to phone the EMS system for help.

2. What do you do next?
   - ☐ a. Check the pulse.
   - ☒ b. Begin rescue breathing.
   - ☐ c. Check for breathing again.

3. How often should you recheck the infant's pulse?
   - ☒ a. After 1 minute and once every minute thereafter
   - ☐ b. After 2 minutes and every 5 minutes thereafter
   - ☐ c. After 4 minutes and every 5 minutes thereafter

You find that there is a pulse but the infant is still not breathing. You continue rescue breathing.

4. How often should you give rescue breaths to an infant?
   - ☐ a. Give 1 breath every second
   - ☒ b. Give 1 breath every 3 seconds
   - ☐ c. Give 1 breath every 6 seconds

Answers

1. You open the airway by doing the head-tilt/**chin**-lift.
   When you check for breathing, you look, **listen**, and feel for breathing.
   You check an infant's pulse by pressing gently against the inside of the upper **arm**.

2. **b.** When an infant is not breathing but has a pulse, you **begin rescue breathing**.

3. **a.** You should recheck the infant's pulse **after 1 minute and once every minute thereafter**.

4. **b.** For an infant, you **give 1 rescue breath every 3 seconds**.

Review Question: First Aid for a Conscious Infant With an Obstructed Airway

You are feeding your 10-month-old nephew. A loud noise scares him just as he has taken a spoonful of food, and he chokes. He cannot cry, cough, or breathe. You shout for help and have someone call the EMS system. What type of first aid should you give?

1. ☐ a. 5 chest compressions followed by 5 rescue breaths
   ☒ b. 4 back blows followed by 4 chest thrusts
   ☐ c. 6 to 10 abdominal thrusts followed by a foreign-body check

The infant coughs up the food.

2. You should watch him carefully until ___*EMS*___ personnel arrive.

Answers

1. **b.** If a conscious infant has choked and cannot cry, cough, or breathe, you should give **4 back blows followed by 4 chest thrusts**.

2. When the infant coughs up the food, you should watch him carefully until **EMS** personnel arrive.

Review Question: First Aid for an Unconscious Infant With an Obstructed Airway

You are watching TV and eating popcorn with a 10-year-old. His 8-month-old brother is crawling near you. You leave the room to answer the phone, and the boy comes running to tell you that there is something wrong with the infant. You find the infant lying on the floor, not moving.

You check for unresponsiveness. He is unconscious. You position him on his back.

1. What should you do next?
   - ☒ a. Open the airway and check for breathing.
   - ☐ b. Give 4 back blows and 4 chest thrusts.
   - ☐ c. Give 1 rescue breath every 3 seconds.

You cannot breathe air into the infant when you give 2 slow breaths.

2. What should you do now?
   - ☐ a. Do a foreign-body check.
   - ☐ b. Give 6 to 10 abdominal thrusts.
   - ☒ c. Retilt the head and give 2 more slow breaths.

You still can't breathe air into the infant.

3. What should you do?
   - ☒ a. Give 4 back blows followed by 4 chest thrusts.
   - ☐ b. Give 6 to 10 abdominal thrusts.
   - ☐ c. Do a foreign-body check.

When doing a foreign-body check, you see an object in the infant's throat and remove it with a finger sweep.

4. What should you do next?
   - ☐ a. Check for a pulse.
   - ☒ b. Give 2 slow breaths.
   - ☐ c. Continue back blows and chest thrusts.

Answers

1. a. If the infant is unconscious, you should **open the airway, and check for breathing**.

2. c. You should **retilt the head and give 2 more slow breaths** if you can't breathe air into the infant.

3. a. If you still can't breathe air into the infant, you should **give 4 back blows followed by 4 chest thrusts**.

4. b. After the object is removed, you should **give 2 slow breaths**.

Review Question: CPR for an Infant

You are at a family cookout with a lot of adults and their children. An older boy runs in and says that his baby sister has fallen into the swimming pool. You rush into the yard and take the infant out of the pool. You check for unresponsiveness and find that she is unconscious.

1. What should you do now?
   - ☒ a. Check the ABCs.
   - ☐ b. Give back blows and chest thrusts.
   - ☐ c. Begin CPR.

You find that the infant is not breathing. You give 2 slow breaths. Then you check the brachial pulse in the upper arm for 5 to 10 seconds. You do **not** feel a pulse.

2. What should you do?
   - ☐ a. Give 1 rescue breath every 3 seconds.
   - ☒ b. Begin CPR.
   - ☐ c. Retilt the head and give 2 more breaths.

3. At what rate should you give chest compressions when doing CPR on an infant?
   - ☐ a. 50 to 60 compressions per minute
   - ☐ b. 70 to 80 compressions per minute
   - ☒ c. At least 100 compressions per minute

4. What is the ratio of compressions to breaths when giving CPR to an infant?
   - ☐ a. 2 compressions to 2 breaths
   - ☒ b. 5 compressions to 1 breath
   - ☐ c. 10 compressions to 2 breaths

5. How far should you compress an infant's chest when giving CPR?
   - ☒ a. ½ to 1 inch (1.3 to 2.5 centimeters)
   - ☐ b. 1½ to 2 inches (2.5 to 3.8 centimeters)
   - ☐ c. 2½ to 3 inches (5.1 to 6.3 centimeters)

After doing 10 cycles (about 1 minute) of continuous CPR, you recheck the infant's pulse for 5 seconds. There is no pulse.

6. What should you do?
   - ☐ a. Give 1 rescue breath every 4 seconds.
   - ☒ b. Continue CPR.
   - ☐ c. Keep the infant warm.

Answers

1. **a.** You should **check the ABCs** if the infant is unconscious.

2. **b.** You should **begin CPR** if the infant is not breathing and has no pulse.

3. **c.** When doing CPR on an infant, you should give compressions at the rate of **at least 100 compressions per minute**.

4. **b.** When giving CPR to an infant, the ratio is **5 compressions to 1 breath**.

5. **a.** When giving CPR to an infant, you should compress the infant's chest **½ to 1 inch** (1.3 to 2.5 centimeters).

6. **b.** If there is no pulse when you recheck for pulse you should **continue CPR**.

Appendixes

The disease that causes most heart attacks can also cause stroke. When one of the vessels carrying blood to or through the brain bursts or becomes blocked by a clot, death to a part of the brain may result. If blood cannot get through to part of the brain, that part of the brain will not get enough oxygen and the brain cells will begin to die (**Fig. 103**). This is called a **stroke**. A stroke is similar to a heart attack, only it happens in the brain. As with a heart attack, your role is to recognize the signals and to take immediate action. This appendix describes those signals and discusses the actions you should take when someone suffers a stroke.

Objectives

By the time you finish reading this appendix, you should be able to do the following:

1. Describe the process that causes a stroke.
2. List three signals of a stroke.
3. Describe the first aid for a stroke.

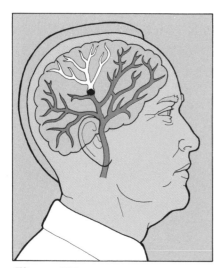

Figure 103
Stroke

Signals of a Stroke

Like the signals of a heart attack, the signals of a stroke may not be easy to recognize. Signals of a stroke may last from seconds to a few minutes to a few hours. The signals that you see will depend on the location of the damaged blood vessel and the amount of damage to the brain. The victim may show one or more of the following signals:
- Sudden, temporary weakness or numbness of the face, arm, or leg on one side of the body.
- Temporary loss of speech, or trouble speaking or understanding speech.
- Temporarily dimmed vision, or loss of vision, particularly in one eye.
- Unexplained dizziness, unsteadiness, or sudden falls.
- Severe headache.

First Aid for Stroke

Here are the steps you should follow when someone suffers a stroke:
1. Recognize the signals of a stroke and take action.
2. Have the victim stop what he or she is doing and rest in a comfortable position.
3. Do not let the victim eat or take medication.
4. Call the EMS system for help.

A key factor in whether or not a victim will survive a stroke is how quickly the victim receives advanced emergency medical care. Therefore, it is important that you call the EMS system right away.

Not all ambulances are staffed and equipped to provide advanced emergency medical care to the victim at the scene of an emergency, but in most cases it is better to call for an ambulance to transport the victim, rather than to transport the victim in a private vehicle yourself. The victim's condition could worsen on the way to the hospital, and an ambulance is equipped and staffed to deal with conditions that could develop during the transport. In addition, transporting a victim in a private vehicle places tremendous emotional pressures on the driver. This puts **all** occupants of the vehicle at added risk.

There may be some situations, however, when an ambulance is not readily available, and you may have to weigh the risks and consider driving the victim to the hospital. You should know that not all hospitals and health facilities offer advanced care. Of those that do, not all offer it on a 24-hour basis. Therefore, it is important to be familiar with the emergency resources of your community and make a plan of action **before** an emergency happens.

After the EMS system has been called, you should ask the victim for information about his or her condition, as explained in Chapter 1. If the victim cannot answer, try to get the information from bystanders.

You should try to learn—

- The victim's name.
- The victim's age.
- The victim's previous medical problems and if anything like this ever happened to the victim before.

If the victim becomes unconscious, position the victim on his or her back and monitor airway, breathing, and circulation. Should the victim vomit, turn his or her head and body to the side and quickly wipe the material out of the mouth. Keeping the victim positioned on his or her side, tilt the head back and monitor airway, breathing, and circulation.

Because the stroke victim's breathing and heart may stop, you should be prepared to give rescue breathing or CPR.

Review Questions

Check the best answer(s) or fill in the blanks with the right word.

1. What happens when a person has a stroke?
    - ☐ a. The flow of blood to part of the heart is blocked.
    - ☐ b. The flow of blood to part of the brain is blocked.
    - ☐ c. The flow of blood to the hands and feet is blocked.

2. What are three signals of a stroke?
    - ☐ a. Temporary loss of speech
    - ☐ b. Weakness or numbness on one side of the body
    - ☐ c. Crushing chest pain
    - ☐ d. Severe headache

3. What is the first aid for a stroke?
    - a. _____ the signals and take action.
    - b. Have the victim _____ in a comfortable position.
    - c. Do not let the victim _____ or take _____.
    - d. Phone the _____ system for help.

Answers

1. **b.** When a person has a stroke, **the flow of blood to part of the brain is blocked.**

2. Three signals of a stroke are—
    a. **Temporary loss of speech.**
    b. **Weakness or numbness on one side of the body.**
    d. **Severe headache.**

3. The first aid for a stroke is—
    a. **Recognize** the signals and take action.
    b. Have the victim **rest** in a comfortable position.
    c. Do not let the victim **eat** or take **medication.**
    d. Phone the **EMS** system for help.

What Is an Emergency Medical Services (EMS) System?

To save a life in a life-threatening situation, two things must happen. Emergency care must be started right away by a trained bystander, and this care must be continued and enhanced by EMS personnel when they arrive. If no one with first aid training is nearby to begin emergency care immediately, or if the community's EMS system cannot quickly provide the right kind of help, then a victim's chances of survival may be greatly reduced.

By taking this course, you have already taken one step to improve the ability of your community's EMS system to save lives. You have increased the chances that a trained person—you—may be able to help at the scene of an accident or other medical emergency until EMS personnel arrive. Your ability to provide care immediately could save a life.

Components of an EMS System

Providing the victim with the right care at the right time is not an easy task. Although most communities have some way of sending medical help to victims of sudden illness or accidents, this help may not include everything that the victim needs and may not arrive in time to give the victim the best chance of surviving. Your community's ability to get the right help to the victim as quickly as possible requires both planning and resources. Effective EMS systems usually have the following parts:
1. **Trained citizens.** Trained citizens like you can give first aid and alert the EMS system that a medical emergency has happened.
2. **Trained personnel.** To provide the best help quickly, an EMS system has specially trained personnel. These may include emergency medical technicians (EMTs), emergency medical technician-paramedics (paramedics), first responders (police, firefighters), emergency dispatchers, and hospital emergency department physicians and nurses trained in emergency medicine.
3. **Special equipment.** Specialized medical, rescue, and transportation equipment is required for various situations.
4. **Communications systems.** How well the EMS system works depends on how quickly citizens can alert the system that an emergency has happened and how quickly the EMS dispatcher can get the appropriate emergency personnel to the scene. Communications systems are also important because EMS personnel often need to communicate with the hospital emergency department as they care for the victim at the scene of the emergency and on the way to the hospital.

Throughout this course, you have learned how important it is for you and your community's EMS system to work together to give the victim of a medical emergency the best chance of survival.

This appendix explains what an EMS system is and how a victim of injury or sudden illness "enters" the system. It also explains the different types of care that a victim may require (basic life support and advanced life support) and what should happen when EMS personnel arrive at the scene of an emergency. At the end of this appendix there is a list of questions to help you learn more about your community's EMS system.

Objectives

By the time you finish reading this appendix, you should be able to do the following:

1. Describe the purpose of an Emergency Medical Services (EMS) system.

2. List at least three parts of an EMS system.

3. Describe the three main responsibilities of a trained citizen-rescuer when a medical emergency occurs.

4. List five facts that you should know about your community's EMS system.

5. **Management and evaluation.** An EMS system needs a management structure that includes administration and coordination of all parts of the system, medical supervision and direction, and ongoing evaluation and research.

The Responsibilities of the Rescuer in the EMS System

In order for the victim of a medical emergency to receive care from the EMS system, the victim must **enter** the system. This means that the EMS system must be told about the emergency. Then, until EMS personnel arrive, the victim should receive the proper first aid. These important first steps are generally performed by a citizen-rescuer. There are three things that **you** must do to make sure that a victim enters the EMS system with the best chance for survival:

1. **Recognize that a medical emergency has happened.** This isn't always easy. For example, you learned in Chapter 4 that victims of heart attack often deny that they are having a heart attack, making it difficult for bystanders to know something is wrong. Also, victims of accidents may be so concerned about the well-being of another injured person that they may not realize that they themselves are hurt. Medical problems are not always obvious, but the skills you have learned in this course will help you recognize emergencies.

2. **Give first aid (basic life support).** You have been trained to provide first aid for breathing and cardiac emergencies. CPR, rescue breathing, and first aid for choking are all basic life support techniques.

3. **Phone the EMS system for help.** You may phone or direct bystanders to phone for help. Give all necessary information so that appropriate medical care can reach the scene of the emergency. This information is discussed in Chapter 1.

How an EMS System Responds to a Call for Help

In many communities, a dispatcher will answer your call. The dispatcher is very important in making sure that the victim gets the right care immediately. In some systems, this person has special training to get specific information from the caller and to know which personnel and equipment to send to the scene. Some dispatchers can also give first aid instructions to the caller over the phone when it is necessary.

Basic Life Support and Advanced Life Support

As explained in Chapter 1, the information you provide to the EMS dispatcher is important. It will help determine the type of care that the dispatcher sends to the scene of an emergency. The dispatcher may send either an ambulance capable of continuing **basic life support** or an ambulance capable of delivering **advanced life support.** The care sent will depend on the needs of the victim and the services available in your community.

Most requests for emergency medical services require basic life support. For this reason, many states require that all ambulances be staffed with personnel trained to provide at least basic life support.

Some requests for assistance also require advanced life support. For example, a victim of a heart attack or cardiac arrest requires both basic life support and advanced life support. Advanced life support personnel may be supervised by a hospital-based physician.

A key thing to remember is that basic life support and advanced life support must be given within specific time periods to give the victim the best chance of survival. This is why it is important to have a well-coordinated EMS system in your community. Highly trained personnel can do more to help the victim if they arrive promptly.

First Responders

When a dispatcher receives a call for emergency medical help, he or she will select the type of care that is needed and send the appropriate personnel. This may include police, fire, rescue, and ambulance personnel, depending on the type of emergency and the resources available at the time of the call.

In many communities, police and firefighters may arrive at the scene before the ambulance because they are often located closer to the scene of the emergency. If you have been caring for a victim, the "first responder" may take over or ask you to assist. On the other hand, the first responder may tell you to continue care while he or she attends to other problems at the scene. It is important that you do not stop caring for a victim until the first responder takes over. You should expect the first responder to ask you for information about the victim. Information that you have gained from the primary and secondary surveys of the victim may be valuable to first responders, EMTs, paramedics, and to the hospital staff who will care for the victim later.

When the Ambulance Arrives

When the ambulance arrives, the EMTs or paramedics will take over responsibility for care of the victim and will provide additional medical care. Their goal is to begin to stabilize the victim's condition (correct life-threatening problems) at the scene. Once this has been done, the EMS personnel will prepare the victim for transport to the appropriate hospital emergency department, and they will continue caring for the victim on the way. When the ambulance arrives at the hospital, the EMS personnel will transfer responsibility for care of the victim to the emergency department staff.

You and Your EMS System

As you can see, the process by which you and the EMS system work together to save a life is complex. You should know that many communities do not have EMS systems that contain all of the features described above.

If you have ever been concerned about someone close to you having a heart attack or being the victim of a medical emergency, you owe it to yourself to find out what type of care your community's EMS system can provide **before** an emergency happens. When minutes count, your knowledge of your community's EMS system can help you make the right decisions. The following checklist has been included to help you find out more about your community's EMS system.

A Guide to Assessing Your Community's Emergency Medical Services (EMS) System

The following questions reflect the EMS standards set forth in the Emergency Medical Services Systems Act of 1973, the federal EMS legislation.

1. Are regularly scheduled CPR and first aid classes, open to the public, offered in your community? Yes____ No____

2. Does your community have a 911 emergency number for EMS, fire, and police? Yes____ No____

3. Do your local schools certify students in first aid and CPR? Yes____ No____

4. Are local police officers trained and certified in American Red Cross First Aid or in the U.S. Department of Transportation First Responder training? Yes____ No____

5. Is your local ambulance service staffed by EMTs? Yes____ No____

6. Does your local ambulance service regularly leave the station to answer an emergency call within two minutes of receiving the call? Yes_____ No_____

7. Does your community have advanced life support units staffed by emergency medical technician-paramedics? Yes_____ No_____

8. Are rescue services in your community (EMS, police, fire) provided by well-equipped units staffed by EMTs? Yes_____ No_____

9. Are all emergency services in your community dispatched and coordinated through a central emergency communications center? Yes_____ No_____

10. Is your nearest hospital emergency department staffed on a 24-hour basis by physicians and nurses who are specially trained in emergency medicine? Yes_____ No_____

11. Does your community have a plan to transfer acutely ill or badly injured patients to specialty centers? Yes_____ No_____

12. Does your community have an area-wide disaster plan to deal with multi-casualty incidents, natural disasters, and environmental emergencies? Yes_____ No_____

13. Is there one office in charge of the administration, coordination, and evaluation of the EMS system? Yes_____ No_____

Adapted from *A Community Scoring Guide for Emergency Health Services*, Office of Emergency Medical Services, The Pennsylvania State University.

With a better idea of the different parts and responsibilities of a community emergency medical services system, you will be better able to assess the emergency medical services offered by your own community.

Your answers to the preceding questions will help you evaluate the services that your community provides. The questions to which you have answered "Yes" will show you the strengths of your community's EMS system. The questions to which you have answered "No" will point out areas where your community's EMS system could be strengthened. As a citizen and a taxpayer, your support of your community's EMS system is as important as your knowing how to perform first aid.

Home Safety Checklist

Use this checklist to spot dangers in your home. When you read each question, mark the "Yes" box if your answer is "yes." Mark the "No" box if your answer is "no." Each mark in a "No" box shows a possible danger for you and your family. Work with your family to remove dangers and make your home safer.

Yes	No	
		Outside the home
☐	☐	Is trash kept in tightly covered containers?
☐	☐	Are walkways, stairs, and railings in good repair?
☐	☐	Are walkways and stairs free of toys, tools, etc.?
☐	☐	Are sandboxes, wading pools, etc. covered when not in use?
		Kitchen
☐	☐	Are pot handles turned inward when cooking?
☐	☐	Are hot dishes kept away from edge of table or counter?
☐	☐	Are hot foods and liquids kept out of child's reach?
☐	☐	Are knives and other sharp items kept out of child's reach?
☐	☐	Is high chair placed away from stove or other hot appliances?
☐	☐	Are matches and lighters kept out of child's reach?
☐	☐	Are all appliance cords kept out of child's reach?
☐	☐	Are cabinets equipped with safety latches?
☐	☐	Are cabinet doors kept closed when not in use?
☐	☐	Are cleaning products kept out of child's reach?
		Bathroom
☐	☐	Are the toilet seat and lid kept down when not in use?
☐	☐	Are cabinets equipped with safety latches?
☐	☐	Are cabinet doors closed when not in use?
☐	☐	Are all medicines in child-resistant containers?
☐	☐	Are all medicines stored in a locked medicine cabinet?
☐	☐	Are shampoos and cosmetics stored out of child's reach?
☐	☐	Are razors, razor blades, and other sharp objects kept out of child's reach?
☐	☐	Are hairdryers and other appliances stored away from sink, tub, and toilet?
☐	☐	Does the bottom of tub or shower have rubber stickers or a rubber mat to prevent slipping?

Yes	No	
		### Child's room
☐	☐	Is child's bed or crib placed away from radiators or other heated surfaces?
☐	☐	Are crib slats no more than 2⅜ inches apart?
☐	☐	Does mattress fit sides of crib snugly?
☐	☐	Is paint on furniture nontoxic?
☐	☐	Are electric cords kept out of child's reach?
☐	☐	Does toy box have a safety hinge or cover?
☐	☐	Are toys in good repair?
☐	☐	Do toys have nontoxic finishes?
☐	☐	Are toys appropriate for the child's age?
☐	☐	Is child's clothing, especially sleepwear, flame resistant?
		### Parent's bedroom
☐	☐	Are space heaters kept away from curtains and flammable materials?
☐	☐	Are cosmetics stored out of child's reach?
		### Storage areas
☐	☐	Are pesticides, detergents, and other household chemicals kept out of child's reach?
☐	☐	Are tools kept out of child's reach?
		### General precautions inside the home
☐	☐	Are stairways kept clear and uncluttered?
☐	☐	Are stairs and hallways well lit?
☐	☐	Are safety gates installed at tops and bottoms of stairways?
☐	☐	Are rugs and runners skidproof?
☐	☐	Are guards installed around fireplaces, radiators or hot pipes, and wood-burning stoves?
☐	☐	Are sharp edges of furniture cushioned with corner guards or other material?
☐	☐	Are unused electric outlets covered with tape or outlet covers?
☐	☐	Are curtain cords and shade pulls kept out of child's reach?
☐	☐	Are windows secured with window locks?
☐	☐	Are plastic bags kept out of child's reach?
☐	☐	Are fire extinguishers installed where they are most likely to be needed?
☐	☐	Are smoke detectors in working order?
☐	☐	Do you have an emergency exit plan to use in case fire?

Yes	No	
☐	☐	Does your family practice using this emergency exit plan?
☐	☐	Is thermostat on water heater set to 120° F?
☐	☐	If you have a firearm, is it locked up where your child cannot get it?
☐	☐	Are all handbags, including those of visitors, kept out of child's reach?.
☐	☐	Are all poisonous plants kept out of child's reach?
☐	☐	Is a list of instructions and important emergency phone numbers posted near phone?
☐	☐	Is a list of instructions posted near phone for use by children who are home alone?
☐	☐	Do you have syrup of ipecac in your home for use as directed in poisoning emergencies?

Glossary

Abdominal thrust—an upward push to the abdomen given to clear the airway of a person with a complete airway obstruction. Also called the Heimlich maneuver.

Adam's apple—the protruding part in the front of the neck formed by the thyroid cartilage. To find the carotid pulse, you must first find the Adam's apple.

Air exchange—the process of respiration, or breathing; inhalation and exhalation of air into and out of the lungs.

Airway—the passageway through which air enters the body and goes to the lungs.

Airway obstruction—a partial or complete blockage of the airway. See **anatomic obstruction** and **mechanical obstruction.**

Anatomic obstruction—blockage of the airway by the tongue or by tissues of the throat.

Arteries—the blood vessels that carry blood away from the heart to the cells of the body.

Artificial respiration—see **rescue breathing.**

Back blow—blow delivered with the heel of your hand between the shoulder blades of an infant. It is used along with chest thrusts to give first aid to an infant who is choking.

Brachial pulse—the beat that is felt on the inside of an infant's upper arm. It is checked to determine the presence or absence of heartbeat. See **pulse.**

Blockage—see **airway obstruction** and **mechanical obstruction.**

Blood pressure—the force of the circulating blood pushing against the walls of the blood vessels.

Blood vessels—the tubes through which blood circulates throughout the body.

Breastbone—the main bone in the front, center part of the chest to which the ribs are connected.

Breathlessness—the absence of breathing.

Cardiac arrest—the condition in which the heart stops beating. CPR must be given promptly to a victim of cardiac arrest to keep blood flowing to the brain and cells of the body.

CPR—the abbreviation for cardiopulmonary resuscitation.

Cardiac emergency—a life-threatening condition in which the heart is not functioning properly, such as a heart attack or cardiac arrest.

Cardiopulmonary resuscitation (CPR)—an emergency procedure used for a person who is not breathing and whose heart has stopped beating (cardiac arrest). The procedure involves a combination of rescue breathing and chest compressions.

Cardiovascular disease—the disease characterized by the gradual clogging of blood vessels by fatty substances. It is associated with heart attacks, strokes, high blood pressure, and diabetes.

Carotid pulse—the beat that is felt at the side of the neck when the carotid artery is pressed. Located between the windpipe and the neck muscle, the carotid pulse is checked to determine the presence or absence of heartbeat. See **pulse.**

Chest compression—a procedure for manually circulating blood in a person whose heart has stopped beating. It involves pressing down and up on the lower half of breastbone. CPR is the combination of chest compressions and rescue breathing.

Chest thrust—a thrust to the middle of the breastbone that is used to clear the airway. It is used for an adult with complete airway obstruction who is extremely overweight or in the late stages of pregnancy. Chest thrusts are also used to give first aid to an infant who is choking.

Child—someone one through eight years old (for the purposes of this course).

Cholesterol—a fatty substance that builds up on the walls of arteries. It is a major contributor to heart disease.

Circulatory emergency—a life-threatening emergency in which the beat of the heart stops or becomes abnormal.

Circulatory system—the system that carries blood to all the cells of the body. Its main components are the blood vessels and the heart.

Glossary

Complete airway obstruction—a condition in which a person is choking and completely unable to breathe, cough, or speak because something is blocking his or her airway.

Decontamination—a thorough cleansing to reduce germs and contaminants.

EMS—the abbreviation for emergency medical services.

EMS dispatcher—a member of the emergency medical services (EMS) system who receives emergency calls and directs the appropriate personnel and equipment to the scene of a medical emergency.

Emergency action principles—the four basic steps to follow in all emergency situations to ensure that victims receive proper care.

Emergency medical services (EMS) system—a community-based system that delivers specialized care for victims who are ill or injured. Care is provided at the scene of the emergency and is continued during transportation and following arrival at an appropriately staffed and equipped health care facility.

Finger pad—the underside of the fingertip. The pads of two fingers are used to compress the breastbone of a choking infant or an infant needing CPR.

Finger sweep—a technique used as part of the procedure to dislodge and remove a piece of food or an object from the airway of an unconscious choking victim.

Foreign body—an object that lodges in a person's airway, causing an obstruction or blockage of the airway.

Foreign-body check—a procedure to determine if an object is lodged in an unconscious child's or infant's airway. If the object is visible, an attempt is made to remove it using the finger sweep.

Head-tilt/chin-lift—a technique used to open the airway of an unconscious person. It is done by applying backward pressure on the forehead and lifting the jaw. This tilts the head back and lifts the chin.

Heart attack—a condition in which blood flow to part of the heart is blocked, causing that part of the heart muscle to die from lack of oxygen.

Heimlich maneuver—see **abdominal thrust.**

High blood pressure—a condition in which the pressure of the blood pumping in the circulatory system is higher than normal. This condition is related to cardiovascular disease.

Implied consent—a legal term used to describe the assumption that an unconscious person, if he or she were conscious, would give consent to a rescuer to provide first aid. When the victim is an unconscious or severely injured child or infant, it is assumed that the parent or guardian would consent to first aid.

Infant—someone between birth and one year old.

Infectious disease—a disease that may be transmitted or spread; a contagious disease.

Injury-prevention plan—a plan to reduce the risk of injury to infants and children by removing dangers, giving supervision, and teaching safety.

Manikin—a life-size model of a person used for practicing first aid skills for respiratory and circulatory emergencies.

Mechanical obstruction—an obstruction or blockage of the airway by a foreign object such as a piece of food.

Mouth-to-mouth breathing—a form of rescue breathing in which a rescuer breathes air into the mouth and lungs of a person who is not breathing.

Mouth-to-nose breathing—a form of rescue breathing in which a rescuer breathes air into the nose and lungs of a person who is not breathing. This is done when injuries or other difficulties make it impossible to perform mouth-to-mouth breathing.

Mouth-to-stoma breathing—a form of rescue breathing in which a rescuer breathes air into the stoma and lungs of a person who is not breathing.

Nausea—a feeling of sickness in the stomach with an urge to vomit.

Neutral position—the position in which an infant's head is placed to open the airway.

Neutral-plus position—The range of positions in which a child's head may be placed to open the airway.

Notch—the place where the lower ribs meet the lower end of the breastbone in the center of the chest. Used as a reference point for finding the correct hand position in CPR.

911—a special telephone number used in many communities to give fast, direct connection to police, fire, and emergency medical services.

Obstruction—blockage. See **airway obstruction.**

Oxygen—a gas that the cells of the body need in order to live. The air we breathe contains about 21 percent oxygen.

Oxygen-carrying blood—blood that contains oxygen.

Partial airway obstruction—a partial blockage of the airway that allows some air exchange to occur.

Primary survey—a series of checks to discover conditions that are immediately life threatening to a victim.

Pulmonary—having to do with the lungs.

Pulse—the rhythmic "beat" in an artery. As the heart pumps blood, the walls of the arteries expand and contract, causing a beat or a pulse. This beat or pulse can be felt by pressing on an artery.

Rescue breathing—the process of breathing air into the lungs of a person who has stopped breathing. Also called **artificial respiration.**

Rescuer—a person trained to survey the scene of an emergency, determine the extent of injuries, and provide first aid until EMS personnel arrive.

Respiratory emergency—a condition in which normal breathing is difficult or absent.

Respiratory system—the body system that draws air into the body and expels waste gases. The main parts are the airway and the lungs.

Resuscitation—an effort to artificially restore or provide normal heart and/or lung function.

Risk factors—the conditions and behaviors that increase the likelihood of a person's developing a disease. Some risk factors (age, sex, and heredity) for cardiovascular disease cannot be changed. Others relate to lifestyle and can be changed.

Secondary survey—a series of checks to discover conditions that are not immediately life threatening to a victim, but that may become life threatening if not corrected. These checks are done after life-threatening injuries have been found and cared for.

Stoma—a surgically created opening in the front of the neck through which a person breathes.

Stroke—a condition in which one or more of the blood vessels to the brain becomes clogged or bursts, causing a part of the brain to die from lack of oxygen.

Universal distress signal for choking—an action in which a choking victim grasps at his or her throat to signal that he or she is choking.

Unresponsiveness—a condition in which a person does not react to verbal or physical stimuli.

Index